AROMA BABY

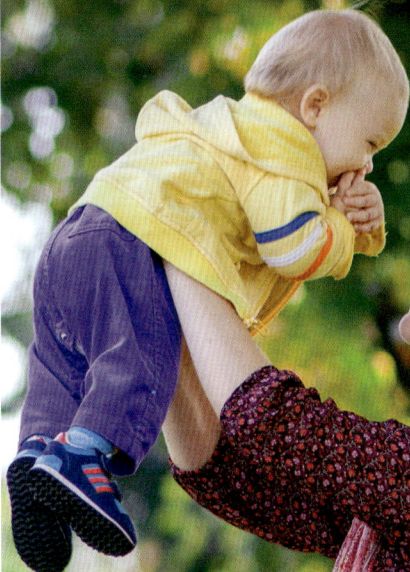

Using Pure Essential Oils During Pregnancy, Childbirth, Infancy, and Early Childhood

LIFE SCIENCE
PRODUCTS & PUBLISHING

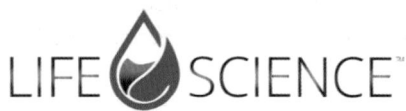

LIFE SCIENCE

Copyright © 2016
Life Science Publishing
1.800.336.6308
www.DiscoverLSP.com

Printed in the United States of America
10 9 8 7 6 5 4 3 2 1

First Printing May 2016 Copyright © 2016 Life Science Publishing www.discoverlsp.com

The information contained in this book is for educational purposes only. It is not provided to diagnose, prescribe, treat, or prevent any condition of the body. The information in this book should not be used as a substitute for medical counseling with a health professional. Neither the author nor publisher accepts responsibility for such use.

Follow all disclaimers and precautions contained in this book. In cases where inflammation may be present, exercise extreme caution in the application of essential oils to the skin. When in doubt, consult a health professional.

FORWARD

Congratulations! If you're reading this book, you or someone close to you is expecting. This is a joyful time—an adventure. If you think about it too much, it could be overwhelming.

But, it doesn't have to be…

Pregnancy and childbirth are a precious time, a loving time. Not everyone gets to experience the joy of conceiving and bearing children. Embrace this time and cherish it. Share the experience with those you love. Know that the sleepless nights, the aches and the pains will be a challenge, but the experience will be worth it.

This book is about learning how to take a more natural approach to your pregnancy. Whether you take a one hundred percent holistic, natural approach, or you combine the best parts of modern medicine with the best parts of traditional, therapeutic essential oils, you have the power to choose. This book is about empowering you to make that choice, to explore information and education associated with complimentary medicine. The approach you choose is up to you.

May you have the best experience and may you and your family experience the greatest joy possible.

Troie Battles

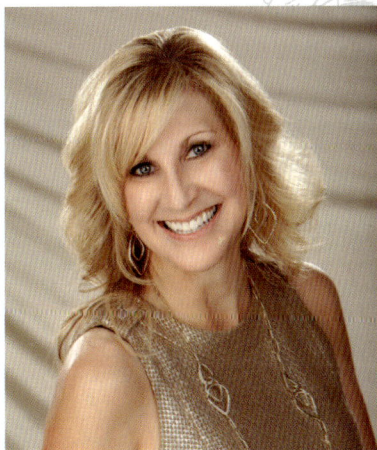

NOTE ABOUT PURITY

It's unfortunate that profit has taken priority over health. All too often, essential oils in the marketplace are diluted with solvents or chemicals. These synthetics and hybrids are not pure, nor are they natural. The essential oils we advocate in the Aroma series are only of the utmost, certified quality. We never advocate a product that may damage health or interfere with healing.

That said, essential oils have been used for thousands of years and have helped countless people to live healthier lives. As publishers of the most sought-after text about essential oils, The Essential Oil Desk Reference, we want to make as much information as easily accessible to you and the people you love.

It is with this spirit of education and sharing that we have compiled and summarized many of the specialized volumes in the Aroma Home series. Always take the time to read, study, and share the things you learn. Use good judgment as you add essential oils into your healthy lifestyle.

As Mary Young has said:

> "Often times, we think we are helping someone by telling them what to do or giving them direction or advice about a problem that person may have. However, we take on a huge responsibility to give advice when we are not the expert or don't have the license that allows us to give advice. Besides that, if we give advice and then that advice doesn't work, that person may become angry with us and can accuse us of 'misdiagnosing, misunderstanding, and wasting their time and money.'

In the world of essential oils, much information is available. If you are going to use any natural product, I suggest that you research all avenues possible and learn as much as you can for yourself, and then you be the one to decide how you will use any particular product.

It doesn't matter what you are going to eat, put on your skin, breathe, or even soak in, learning as much about your product is the most intelligent and safest thing you can do for yourself. The more information you have, the better choices you will make. After you study and research it for yourself, you may decide you don't want the very thing you thought you were excited about; but that is your decision, not someone else's decision about what you should do.

If you find something that interests you and you are uncertain, ask your doctor or someone educated in the field of health and nutrition. Ask their opinion to add to your knowledge bank. Look on the Internet to learn what research institutes, wellness centers, government agencies, the Surgeon General, and even the FDA have to say. You don't have to agree, but it is to your advantage to know what they say.

It is your responsibility to be responsible for yourself. It is your God-given right to search, read, study, and decide how you will feed and take care of your own body. Be independent and be wise."

--- From A Thought From Mary,
   Mary Young 2016

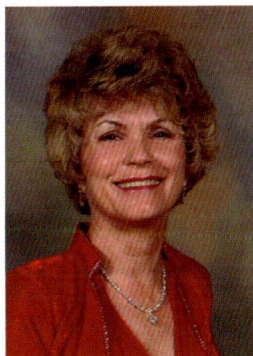

DISCLAIMER

The essential oils and supplemental products discussed at length in this book are the sole product of Young Living. The authors and publisher are completely separate entities from Young Living Essential Oils. Products mentioned may be reformulated, discontinued, expanded, or enhanced by Young Living Essential Oils at any given time.

Neither the authors nor the publisher advocate the use of any other essential oils without the Seed to Seal® guarantee. Even minor changes in the quality of an essential oil may render it, at best, useless and, at worst, dangerous. The use of essential oils during pregnancy, post-partum, infancy, and early childhood should be done with thorough study, watchful care, and judicious prudence.

Many of the suggestions in this book are derived from the *Essential Oils Desk Reference*, one of the most widely sought, sold, and read essential oils books of all time.

TABLE OF CONTENTS

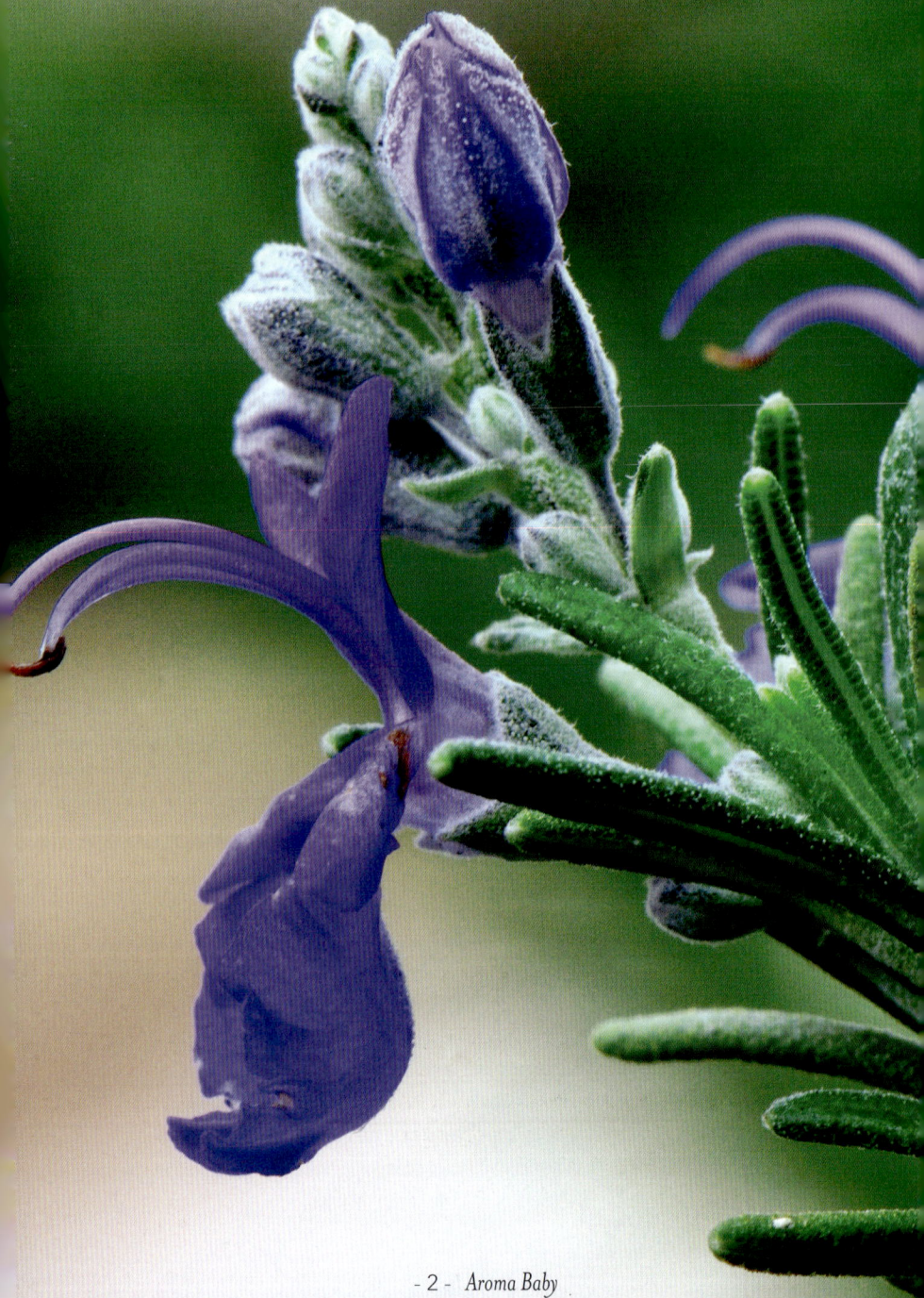

WHAT ARE ESSENTIAL OILS?

Essential oils are the aromatic, volatile liquid you find in many shrubs, flowers, trees, roots, bushes, and seeds. Usually, the best way to extract these liquids is through steam distillation.

Each essential oil is very complex and may consist of hundreds of unique chemical compounds. They are also highly concentrated and far more potent than dried herbs because of the distillation process. So, it takes a lot of plant material to produce tiny amounts of a high quality, distilled essential oil. For example, it takes 5,000 pounds of rose petals to produce 35 ounces of rose oil.

A single essential oil may have as many as 300 or more different constituents that help to make it effective, and the way the oil is distilled or extracted can have dramatic effects on its chemistry and makeup. In some cases, oils that come from a second or third distillation of the same plant material are not as potent as the extracted oils from the first distillation. On the other hand, there are some cases when certain helpful compounds are released only in the second or third distillation.

Why is Purity an Issue?

Excessive heat and pressure can break down delicate aromatic compounds, and this can damage the therapeutic qualities. This means that the steam distillation is a blend of art and science. The best distillers can extract the most ideal profile by paying close attention to temperature, pressure, and duration.

The biggest challenge is knowing that your oil hasn't been diluted with synthetic compounds such as diethylphthalate or dipropylene glycol. Sadly, most of the essential oils you can buy will have traces of dangerous solvents, and these can threaten your health and the health of your baby. That's why you always want the purest, most effective oils.

WAYS OF USING ESSENTIAL OILS

How do you use Essential Oils?

Historically, there were three different models for using essential oils: English, French, and German.

The English model focuses on putting a small amount of an essential oil in a large amount of vegetable oil, mostly for the purpose of massage.

The French model is about applying therapeutic-grade, undiluted (neat) essential oils directly to the skin. This school of thought even recommends taking essential oils internally by adding a few drops to agave nectar, honey, a small amount of vegetable oil, or on a piece of bread.

The German model focuses mainly on inhaling the essential oils for the beneficial effects of fragrance on the brain. Studies show that some essential oils high in sesquiterpenes, such as Young Living's Myrrh, Sandalwood, Cedarwood, Vetiver, and Melissa can dramatically increase oxygenation and activity in the brain, which may directly improve the function of many systems of the body.

Together, these three models show the versatility and power of essential oils. By integrating all three models with various methods of application such as Vita Flex, auricular technique, lymphatic massage, and Raindrop Technique, the best possible results may be obtained.

Three Main Ways to Use Essential Oils

There are three primary ways that you can use essential oils—topical, inhalation, and internally. In some cases, it might be better to inhale the oils. The direct stimulation of the brain can boost mood, concentration, or even stimulate the limbic system.

At other times, it might be better to apply the essential oils topically. This is particularly true for injuries, healing, and relaxation.

When it comes to taking the oils internally, there are a few options. You can add it to vegetable oil, yacon syrup, honey, or a gelatin capsule. We recommend using the Vitality line from Young Living Essential Oils that has specific labeling for internal use.

In some cases, all three ways can be interchangeable and may offer the same benefits. Take Peppermint, for example. A drop or two of Peppermint Vitality™ in a glass of water can be very effective. You might drink Peppermint Vitality™ for indigestion, but you may also get similar results if you were to massage 2-3 drops of regular Peppermint on your abdominal area.

The ability of essential oils to act on both the mind and the body is what makes them truly unique among natural therapeutic substances. The fragrance of some essential oils can be very stimulating—both psychologically and physically. The fragrance of other essential oils may be calming and sedating, helping to overcome anxiety or hyperactivity. On a physiological level, essential oils may stimulate immune function and regenerate damaged tissue. Essential oils may also combat infectious disease by killing viruses, bacteria, and other pathogens.

Diffusing

Probably the two most common methods of essential oil application are cold-air diffusing and neat (undiluted) topical application. Other modes of application include incorporating essential oils into the disciplines of reflexology, Vita Flex, and acupressure. Combining these disciplines with essential oils enhances the healing response and often produces amazing results that cannot be achieved by acupuncture or reflexology alone. Just 1–3 drops of an essential oil applied to an acupuncture meridian or Vita Flex point on the hand or foot can produce results within a minute or two.

The Bible contains over 200 references to aromatics, incense, and ointments. Aromatics such as Frankincense, Myrrh, Galbanum, Cinnamon, Cassia, Rosemary, Hyssop, and Spikenard were used for anointing and healing the sick.

What's in an Essential Oil?

The aromatic constituents of essential oils (i.e., terpenes, monoterpenes, phenols, aldehydes, etc.) are constructed from long chains of carbon and hydrogen atoms, which have a predominantly ring-like structure. Links of carbon atoms form the backbone of these chains, with oxygen, hydrogen, nitrogen, sulfur, and other carbon atoms attached at various points of the chain.

Essential oils have different chemistry than fatty oils (also known as fatty acids). In contrast to the simple linear carbon-hydrogen structure of fatty oils, essential oils have a far more complex ring structure and contain sulfur and nitrogen atoms that fatty oils do not have.

Purity and Potency of Essential Oils

One of the factors that determines the purity of an oil is its constituents. These constituents can be affected by many variables, including the part(s) of the plant from which the oil was produced, soil condition, fertilizer (organic or chemical), geographical region, climate, altitude, harvesting methods, and distillation processes.

The key to producing a therapeutic-grade essential oil is to preserve as many of the delicate aromatic components within the essential oil as possible. Fragile aromatic components are easily destroyed by high temperature and pressure, as well as by contact with reactive metals such as copper or aluminum. This is why all therapeutic-grade essential oils should be distilled in stainless steel cooking chambers at low pressure and low temperature.

The plant material should also be free of herbicides and other chemicals. These can react with the essential oil during distillation to produce toxic compounds. Because many pesticides are oil-soluble, they can also mix into the essential oil.

Although chemists have successfully recreated the main constituents and fragrances of some essential oils in the laboratory, these synthetic oils lack therapeutic benefits and may even carry risks. Pure essential oils contain hundreds of different bioconstituents, which lend important therapeutic properties to the oil when combined. Also, many essential oils contain molecules and isomers that are impossible to manufacture in the laboratory.

Today approximately 300 essential oils are distilled or extracted worldwide. Several thousand constituents and aromatic

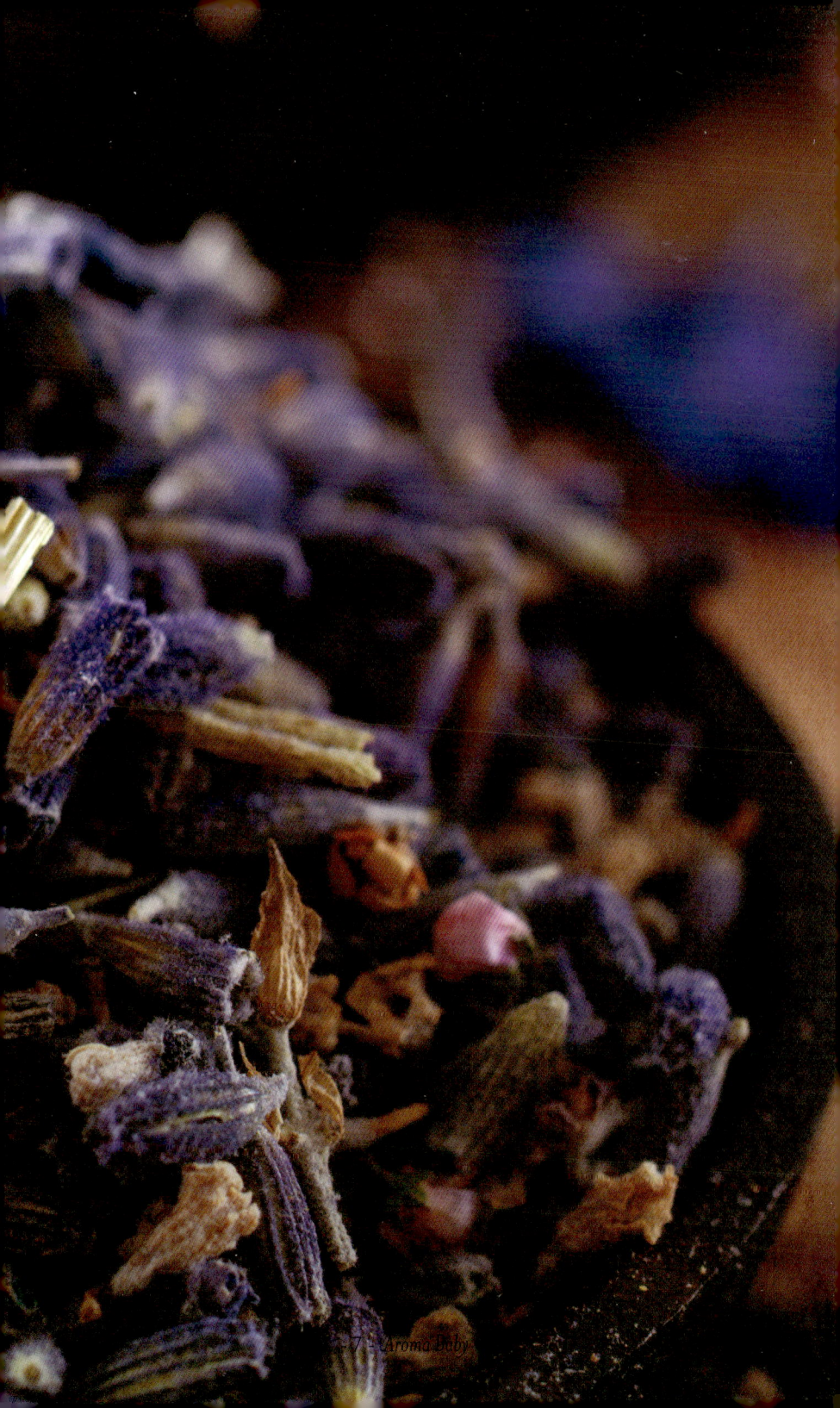

molecules are identified and registered in these 300 essential oils. Ninety-eight percent of essential oil volume produced today is used in the perfume and cosmetic industry. Only about two percent of the production volume is for therapeutic and medicinal applications.

Young Living requires all distillers who want to sell to Young Living to submit samples to be analyzed to ensure that all the constituents are present at the right percentage to be therapeutic. You can have pure oils, but if the plants are distilled at the wrong time of day or with incorrect distillation procedures, the constituents that make the oils therapeutic will not be there, and you will not have a therapeutic-grade profile.

In addition, Young Living requires that the farms and the essential oil distillation facilities be subject to site inspection. Of oil samples submitted between May 2007 and October 2011 by distillers wanting to partner with Young Living, over 34 percent did not meet Young Living standards and were rejected.

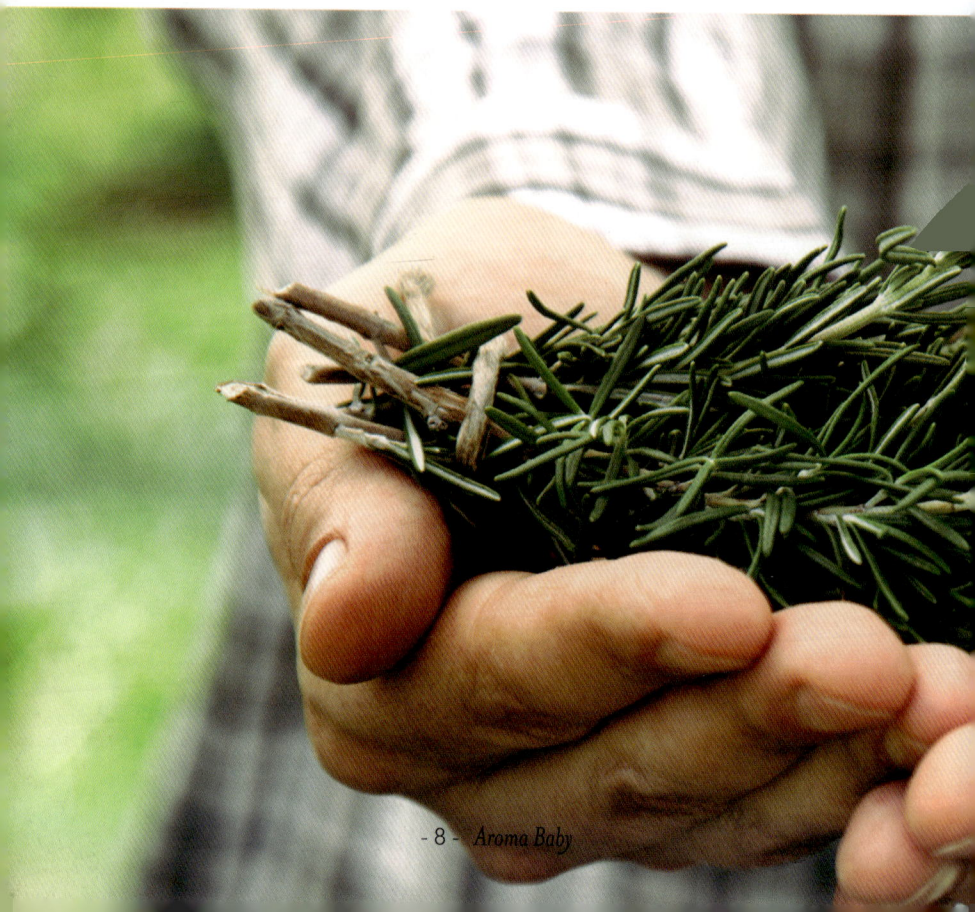

Because Young Living interacts with the end-users who purchase essential oils, the company is able to monitor human response to and determine the actual therapeutic benefit of various oils, thereby comparing the constituents of different oils to determine their maximum, health-giving potential. Quality and efficacy are moving, evolving targets. No one understands this more than Young Living.

STANDARDS AND TESTING

Young Living Standards

Over the years, Young Living has bought and compiled an essential oil retention index and mass spectral reference library that contains over 400,000 components. Using this research reference library, Young Living developed its own standards to guarantee the highest possible therapeutic potency for its essential oils.

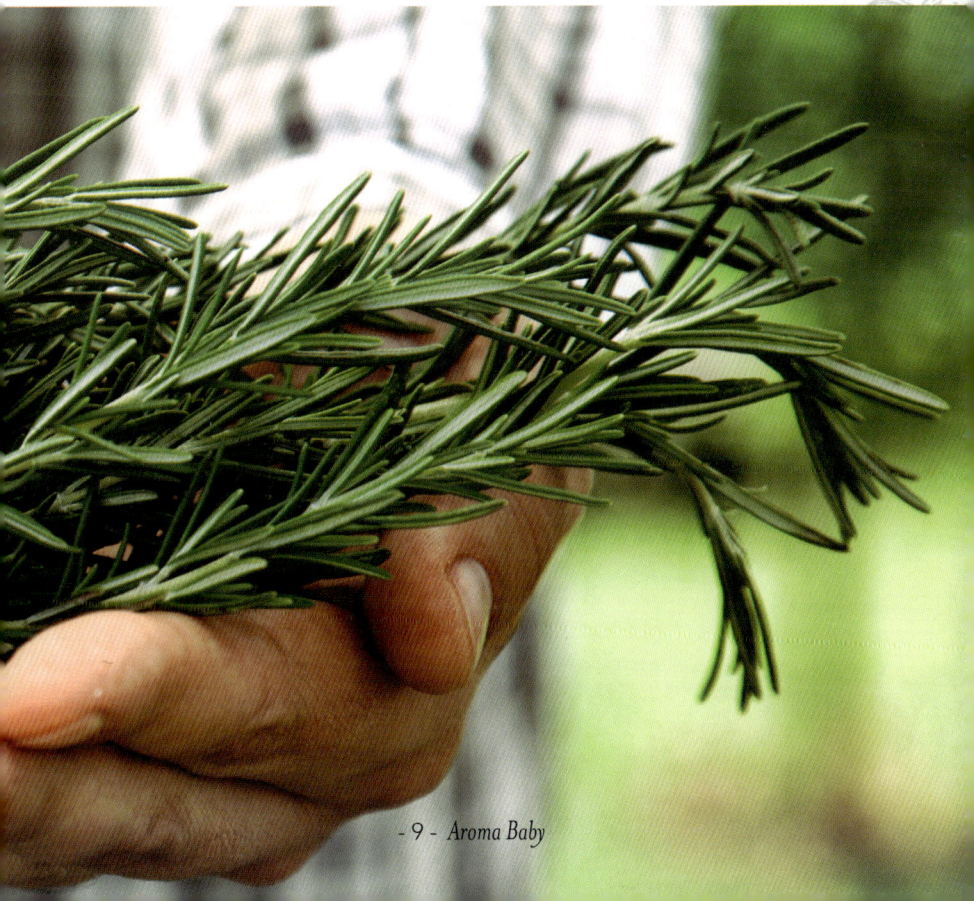

A lavender essential oil produced in one region of France might have a slightly different chemistry than that grown in another region and as a result may not meet the standard. It may have excessive camphor levels (1.0 instead of 0.5), a condition that might be caused by distilling lavender that was too green, or the levels of lavandulol may be too low due to certain weather conditions at the time of harvest.

Adulterated Oils and Their Dangers

Today much of the lavender oil sold in America is a hybrid called lavandin, grown and distilled throughout the world. Lavandin is often heated to evaporate the camphor, mixed with synthetic linalyl acetate to improve the fragrance, and then sold as lavender oil. Most consumers don't know the difference and are happy to buy it for $7 to $10 per half ounce in various stores and on the Internet. This is one of the reasons why it is important to know about the integrity of the essential oil company or vendor.

Adulterated oils that are mixed with synthetic extenders can be very detrimental, causing rashes, burns, and skin irritations. Common additives such as propylene glycol, DEP, or DOP (solvents that have no smell and increase the volume) can cause allergic reactions, besides being devoid of any therapeutic effects.

Some people assume that because an essential oil is "100 percent pure," it will not burn their skin. This is not true. Some pure essential oils may cause skin irritation if applied undiluted. If straight oregano oil is applied to the skin of some people, it may cause severe reddening. Citrus and spice oils like orange and cinnamon may also produce rashes. Even the terpenes in conifer oils like pine may cause skin irritation on sensitive people.

WHY ESSENTIAL OILS WORK

The fragrance of an essential oil can directly affect everything from your emotional state to your lifespan. The specific mechanics of the sense of smell are still being explored by scientists but have been described as working like a lock and key or an odor molecule fitting a specific receptor site.

Because the limbic system is directly connected to those parts of the brain that control heart rate, blood pressure, breathing, memory, stress levels, and hormone balance, essential oils can have profound physiological and psychological effects.

The sense of smell is the only one of the five senses directly linked to the limbic lobe of the brain, the emotional control center. Anxiety, depression, fear, anger, and joy all emanate from this region. The scent of a special fragrance can evoke memories and emotions before we are even consciously aware of it. When smells are concerned, we react first and think later. All other senses (touch, taste, hearing, and sight) are routed through the thalamus, which acts as the switchboard for the brain, passing stimuli onto the cerebral cortex (the conscious thought center) and other parts of the brain.

The limbic lobe (a group of brain structures that includes the hippocampus and amygdala located below the cerebral cortex) can also directly activate the hypothalamus. The hypothalamus is one of the most important parts of the brain. It controls body temperature, hunger, thirst, fatigue, sleep, and circadian cycles. It acts as our hormonal control center and releases hormones that can affect many functions of the body. The production of growth hormones, sex hormones, thyroid hormones, and neurotransmitters such as serotonin are all governed by the hypothalamus.

Essential oils—through their fragrance and unique molecular structure—can directly stimulate the limbic lobe and the hypothalamus, which is responsive to olfactory stimuli. Not only can the inhalation of essential oils be used to combat stress and emotional trauma, but it can also stimulate the production of hormones from the hypothalamus. This results in increased thyroid hormones (our energy hormone) and growth hormones (our youth and longevity hormone).

Grades of Essential Oils

Four grades of essential oils are produced today:

1. **Synthetic or nature-identical oils** (created in a laboratory)

2. **Extended or altered oils** (fragrance grade)

3. **Natural oils and certified oils** (pass oil-standard tests but may not contain any or just a few therapeutic compounds)

4. **Therapeutic-grade essential oils** (pure, medicinal, steam-distilled essential oils containing all desired therapeutic compounds)

Synthetic or nature-identical oils are commonplace in the market and can be created cheaply and then sold in places like health food and drug stores or novelty and tourist shops for a very low price. They have no therapeutic efficacy and may even be harmful. For instance, fragrance-grade lavender may have a harmful effect instead of a healing effect on newly burned skin.

Extended or altered oils may have an essential oil base but are "enhanced" with certain lab-created constituents to increase volume or fragrance. Due to chemical impurities or an antagonistic balance among oil constituents, these oils may be either ineffective or even cause negative effects.

SEED TO SEAL®

Young Living Essential Oils is the only company dedicated to providing 100% therapeutic oils. They are the only company that is able to guarantee essential oil quality from Seed to Seal®.

Years of experience have resulted in knowing the optimum species with the most therapeutic potential and the optimal time and manner to cultivate and harvest them.

Equally important, the freshly distilled oil is filtered, while stringent laboratory testing verifies the potency of the oil and desired chemical structure. The oil is then poured into bottles in Young Living's clean-room facility and shipped.

Young Living's Seed to Seal process guarantees a genuine, pure essential oil that has the highest therapeutic efficacy. This guarantee includes oils distilled from plants grown on Young Living's own farms, sourced from experienced distillers of many generations, or purchased from distillers who have been directed and taught distilling techniques by Gary Young. Young Living's essential oils continue to be used worldwide in more clinical and university studies than any other essential oils today.

Seed
Herbs are selected for the proper genus, species, and chemotype. Whether seeking Clove oil from Madagascar, Cistus oil from Spain, or Helichrysum oil from Corsica, Young Living experts constantly travel across the globe to verify plant, cultivation, and extraction quality to ensure absolute integrity of the essential oil.

Cultivation
Young Living's essential oils are extracted from both wildcrafted and cultivated herbs, from established partnerships with growers and distillers all over the world. Some oils come from herbs cultivated in rural areas of countries such as Madagascar, Indonesia, and Brazil, harvested by indigenous peoples, who have untold years of experience with the plants and their growing conditions. Other oils come from Young Living farms in Ecuador, France, and the United States, where organic practices are adhered to with great care and exactness.

Organic Herb Farming
The key to producing oils with genuine therapeutic quality starts with the proper cultivation of the herbs in the field.

- Plants should be grown on virgin land uncontaminated by chemical fertilizers, pesticides, fungicides, or herbicides. They should also be grown away from nuclear plants, factories, interstates, highways, and heavily populated cities, if possible.

- Because robust, healthy plants produce higher quality essential oils, the soil should be nourished with enzymes, minerals, and organic mulch. The mineral content of the soil is crucial to the proper development of the plant, and soils that lack minerals result in plants that produce inferior oils.

- Land and crops should be watered with deep-well, reservoir, or water-shed water. Mountain stream water is best because of its purity and high mineral content. Municipally treated water or secondary run-off water from residential and commercial areas can introduce undesirable chemical residues into the plant and the essential oil.

- Different varieties of plants produce different qualities of oils. Only those plants that produce the highest quality essential oil should be selected.

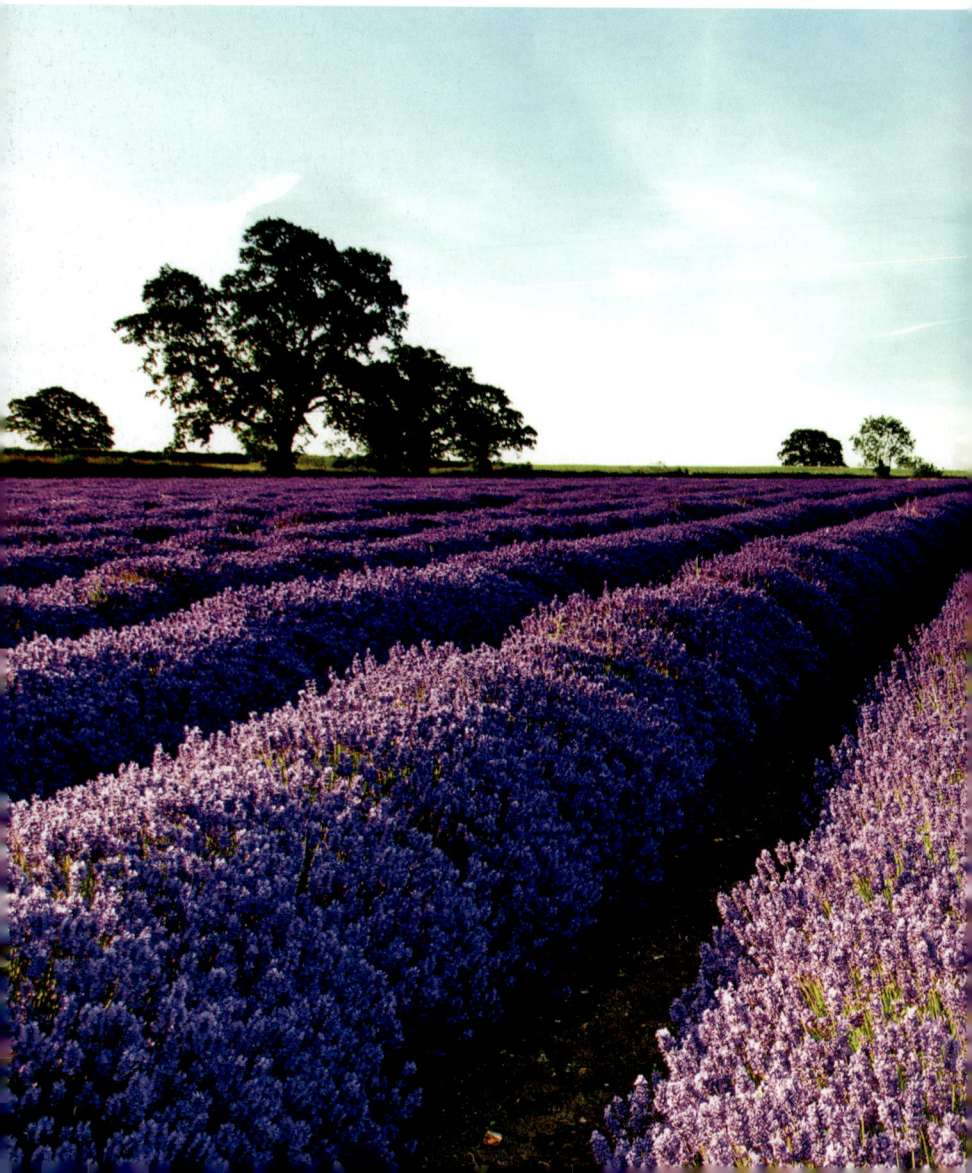

Harvesting

The timing of the harvest is one of the most important factors in the production of therapeutic-grade oils. If the plants are harvested at the wrong time of the season or even at the incorrect time of day, they may distill into a substandard essential oil. In some instances, changing harvest time, by even a few hours, can make a huge difference. For example, German Chamomile harvested in the morning will produce oil with far more azulene (a powerful anti-inflammatory compound) than if it is harvested in the late afternoon.

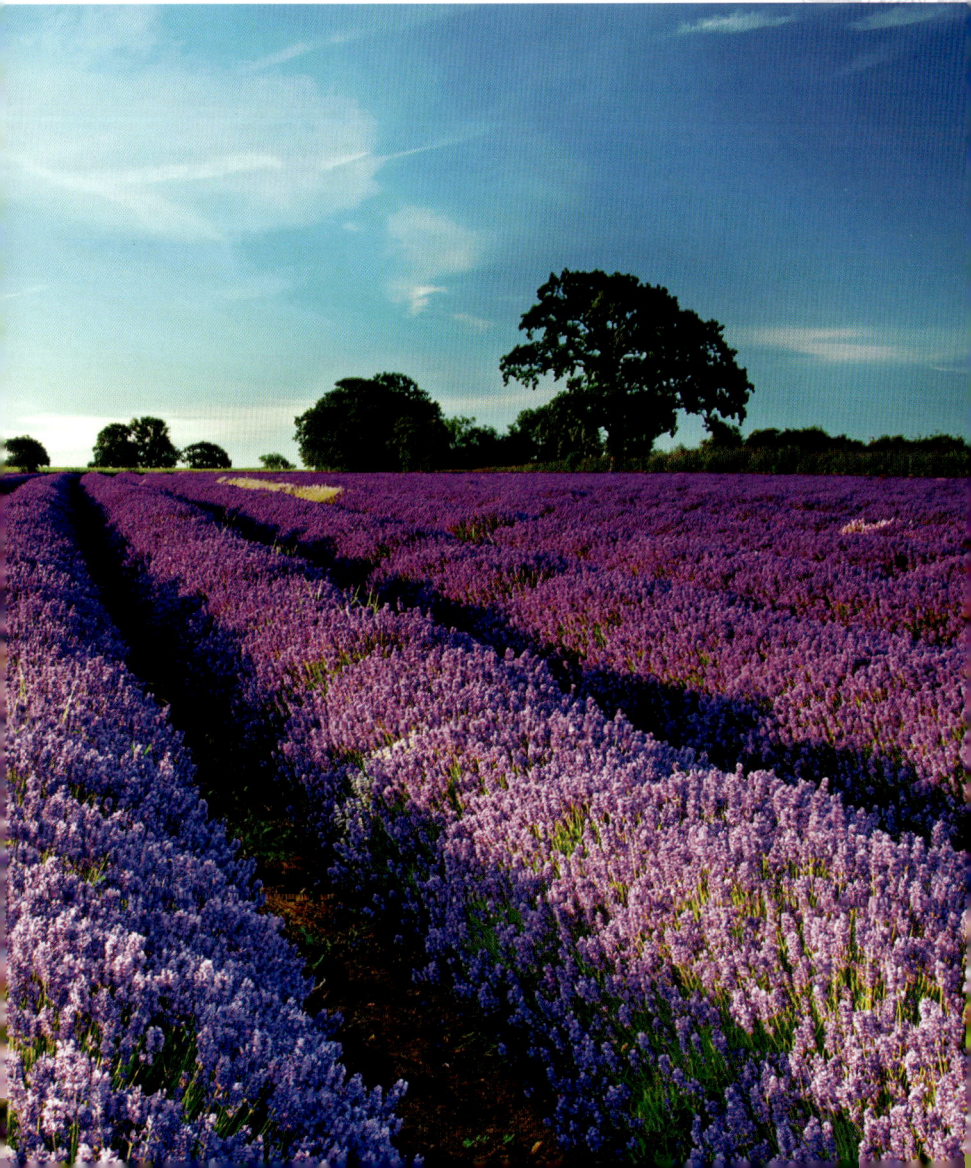

Other factors that should be taken into consideration during the harvest include the amount of dew on the leaves, the percentage of plant in bloom, and weather conditions during the two weeks prior to harvest.

To prevent herbs from drying out prior to being distilled, distillation facilities should be located as close to the field as possible. Transporting herbs to distillation facilities hundreds or thousands of miles away heightens the risk of exposure to pollutants, dust, mold, and petrochemical residues. Young Living continues to expand and develop strategic partnerships with growers and distillers throughout the world.

Different Forms of Essential Oil Production

STEAM DISTILLATION is a separation process for materials that are temperature sensitive like essential oils. Three methods of steam distillation are simple, hydro, and traditional.

In each of these processes as the steam rises, it carries the released oil vapor into the condenser, where the water and oil vapor convert to a liquid and flow into the separator so that the oil can rise to the top of the water and be drained off.

Steam distillation has many variables. Subtle differences in equipment design and processing conditions can translate into huge differences in essential oil quality. The size and material of the extraction chamber, the type of condenser and separator, and the temperature and pressure can all have a huge impact on the oil quality.

EXPRESSED OILS are pressed from the rind of fruits such as Grapefruit, Lemon, Lime, Mandarin, Orange, and Tangerine. Rich in terpene alcohols, expressed oils are not technically "essential oils," even though they are highly regarded for their therapeutic properties and used in the same way as Lavender, Melaleuca, and other essential oils. Expressed oils should be sourced only from organically grown crops, since pesticide residues can become highly concentrated in the oil.

SOLVENT-EXTRACTION involves the use of oil-soluble solvents, such as hexane, di-methylene-chloride, and acetone.

ABSOLUTES are technically not "essential oils" but are "essences." They are obtained from the grain alcohol extraction of a concrete, which is the solid, waxy residue derived from the extraction of plant materials, usually flower petals. This method of extraction is used primarily for botanicals where the fragrance and therapeutic parts of the plant can only be unlocked using solvents. Jasmine and Neroli are extracted this way.

BASIC GUIDELINES FOR SAFE USE

Guidelines are important to follow when using essential oils, especially if you are unfamiliar with the oils and their benefits. Many guidelines are listed here and are elaborated on throughout the book. However, no list of do's and don'ts can ever replace common sense. Start gradually and patiently find what works best for you and your family members.

Storage

1. Always keep a bottle of a pure vegetable oil (e.g., V-6™ Vegetable Oil Complex, olive oil, almond oil, coconut oil, or more fragrant massage oils such as Sensation™, Relaxation™, Ortho Ease™, or Ortho Sport™) handy when using essential oils. Vegetable oils will dilute essential oils if the essential oils cause discomfort or skin irritation.

2. Keep bottles of essential oils tightly closed and store them in a cool location away from light. If stored properly, essential oils will maintain their potency for many years.

3. Keep essential oils out of reach of children. Treat the oils as you would any product for therapeutic use. Children love the oils and will often go through an entire bottle in a very short time. They want to give massages and do the same things they see you do.

Usage

4. Essential oils rich in menthol (such as Peppermint) should not be used on the throat or neck area of children under 18 months of age.

5. Angelica, Bergamot, Grapefruit, Lemon, Orange, Tangerine, and other citrus oils are photosensitive and may cause a rash or dark pigmentation on skin exposed to direct sunlight or UV rays within 1–2 days after application.

6. Keep essential oils away from the eye area and never put them directly into ears. Do not handle contact lenses or rub eyes with essential oils on your fingers. Even in minute amounts, many essential oils may damage contacts and will irritate eyes.

7. Pregnant women should consult a health-care professional when starting any type of health program. Oils are safe to use, but one needs to use common sense. Follow the directions and dilute with V-6 Vegetable Oil Complex until you become familiar with the oils you are using.

    Many pregnant women have said that they feel a very positive response from the unborn child when the oils are applied on the skin, but that is each woman's individual experience.

8. Epileptics and those with high blood pressure should consult their health-care professional before using essential oils. Use extra caution with high ketone oils such as Basil, Rosemary, Sage, and Tansy oils.

9. People with allergies should test a small amount of oil on an area of sensitive skin, such as the inside of the upper arm, for 30 minutes before applying the oil on other areas of the body.

10. The bottoms of feet are safe locations to apply essential oils topically.

11. Direct inhalation of essential oils can be a deep and intensive application method, particularly for respiratory congestion and illness. However, this method should not be used more than 10–15 times throughout the day without consulting a health professional. Also, inhalation of essential oils is NOT recommended for those with asthmatic conditions.

12. Before taking GRAS (Generally Regarded As Safe) essential oils internally, test your reactions by diluting 1 drop of essential oil in 1 teaspoon of an oil-soluble liquid like Blue Agave, Yacon Syrup, olive oil, coconut oil, or rice milk. If you intend to consume more than a few drops of diluted essential oil per day, we recommend first consulting a health professional. Use Young Living's Vitality line for internal consumption and always follow directions listed on the individual bottles

13. Be aware that reactions to essential oils, both topically and Ingestion / Oral, can be delayed as long as 2–3 days.

14. Add 1–3 drops of undiluted essential oils directly to bath water. If more essential oil is desired, mix the oil first into bath salts or a bath gel base before adding to the bath water. Generally, never use more than 10 drops of essential oils in one bath. When essential oils are put directly into bath water without a dispersing agent, they can cause serious discomfort on sensitive skin because the essential oils tend to float, undiluted, on top of the water.

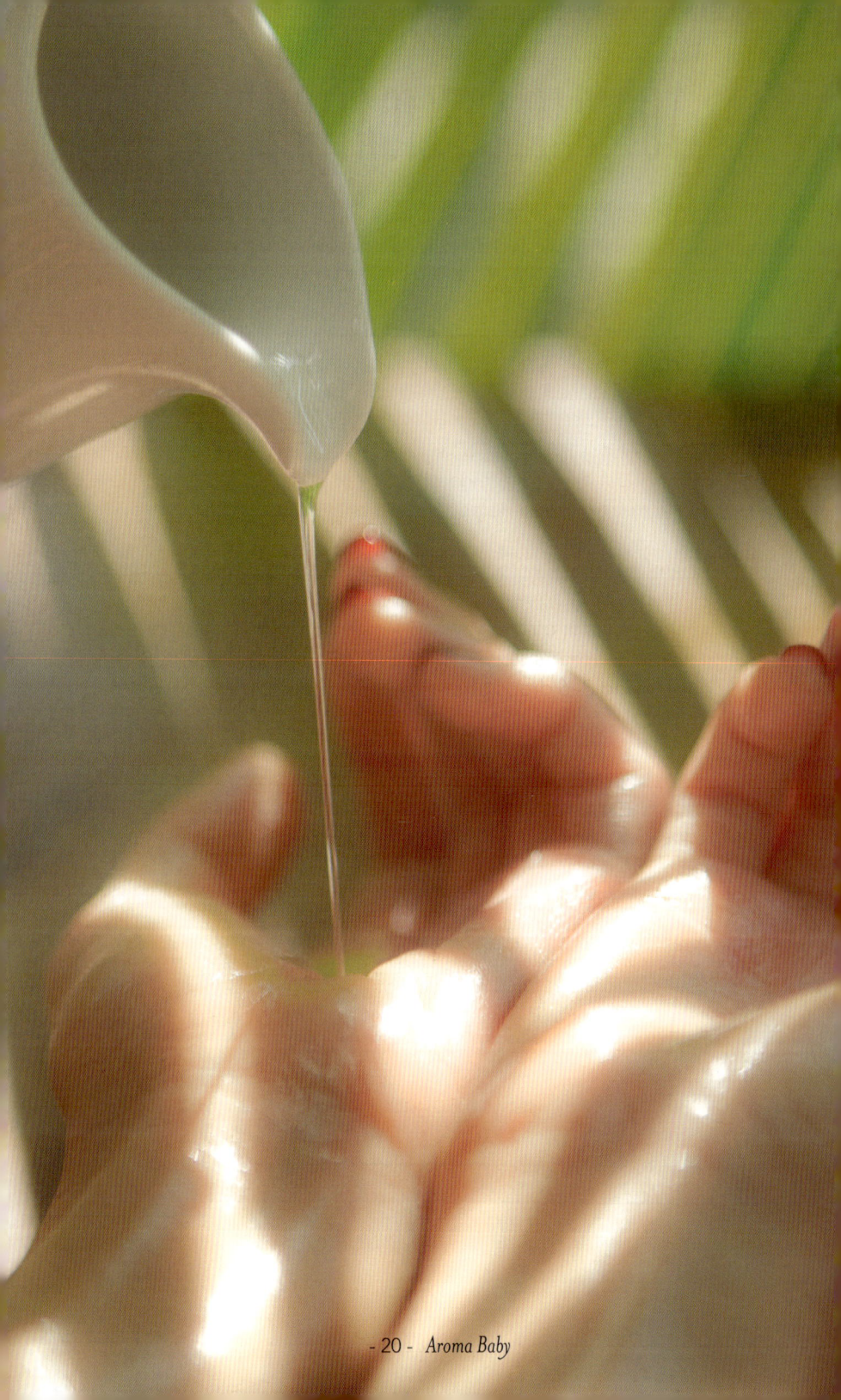

TOPICAL APPLICATION

Many oils are safe to apply directly to the skin. Lavender is safe to use on children without dilution. However, you must be sure the essential oil you are using is not lavandin labeled as lavender or genetically altered lavender. When applying most other essential oils on children, dilute the oils with carrier oil. For dilution, add 15–30 drops of essential oil to 1 oz. of quality carrier oil, as mentioned previously.

Carrier oils such as V-6 Vegetable Oil Complex extend essential oils and provide more efficient use. When massaging, the vegetable oil helps lubricate the skin.

When starting an essential oil application, depending on which oil you use, you may want to test for skin sensitivity by applying the oil first to the bottoms of the feet. See the Vita Flex foot charts to identify areas of best application. Start by applying 3–6 drops of a single oil or blend, spreading it over the bottom of each foot.

When applying essential oils to yourself, use 1–2 drops of oil on 2–3 locations 2 times a day. Increase to 4 times a day if needed. Apply the oil and allow it to absorb for 2–3 minutes before applying another oil or before getting dressed to avoid staining clothing.

As a general rule, when applying oils to yourself or another person for the first time, do not apply more than two single oils or blends at one time. Before applying oils, wash hands thoroughly with soap and water.

When mixing essential oil blends or diluting essential oils in a carrier oil, it is best to use containers made of glass or earthenware, rather than plastic. Plastic particles can leach into the oil and then into the skin once it is applied.

Massage

Start by applying 2 drops of a single oil or blend on the skin and massaging it in. If you are working on a large area, such as the back, mix 1–3 drops of the selected essential oil into 1 teaspoon of pure carrier oil such as V-6 Vegetable Oil Complex, a massage oil, or any other oil of your choice such as jojoba, almond, coconut, olive, and/or grape seed.

Keep in mind that many massage oils such as olive, almond, jojoba, or wheat germ oil may stain some fabrics.

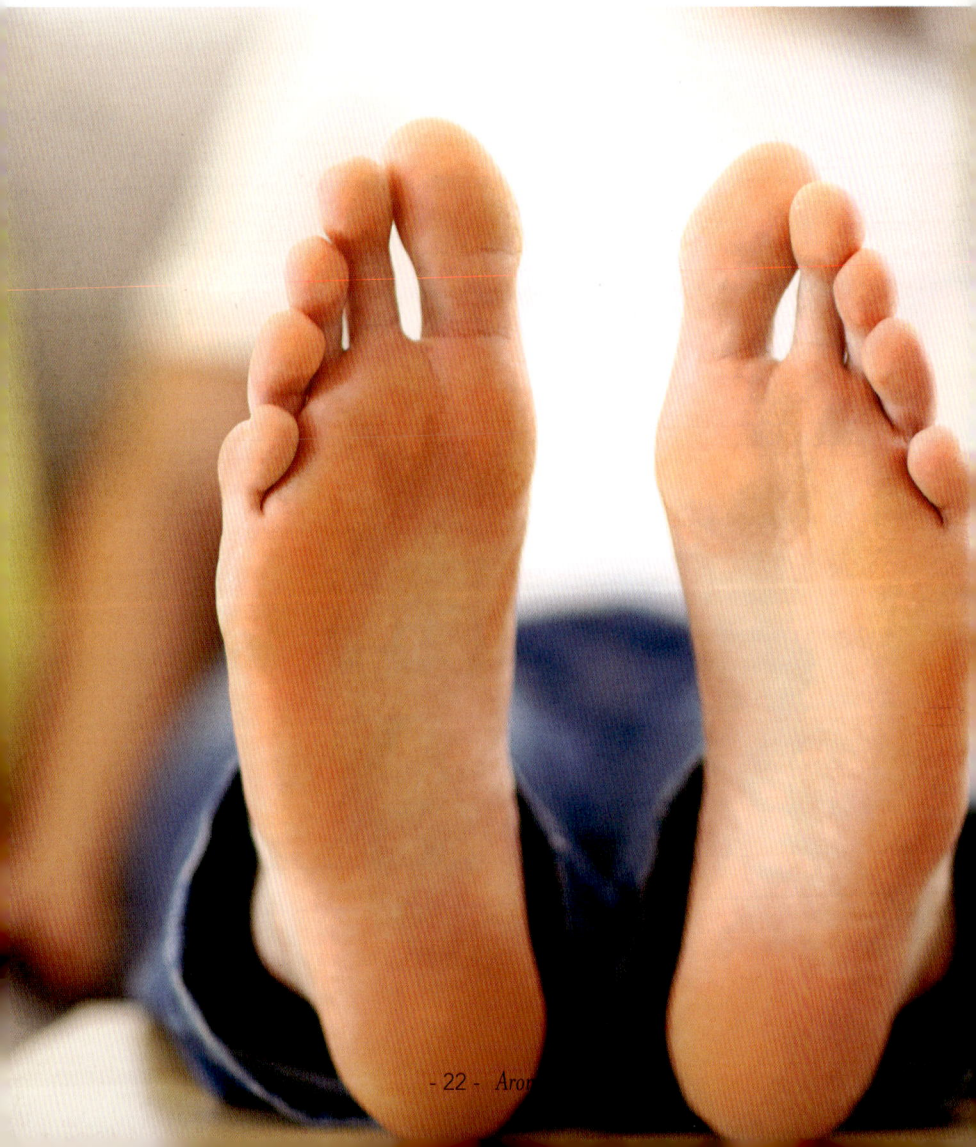

Acupuncture

Licensed acupuncturists can dramatically increase the effectiveness of acupuncture by using essential oils. Talk to your health care provider to discuss how this technique may be beneficial to your pregnancy.

Acupressure

When performing an acupressure treatment, apply 1–3 drops of essential oil to the acupressure point with your finger. Using an auricular probe with a slender point to dispense oil may enhance the application.

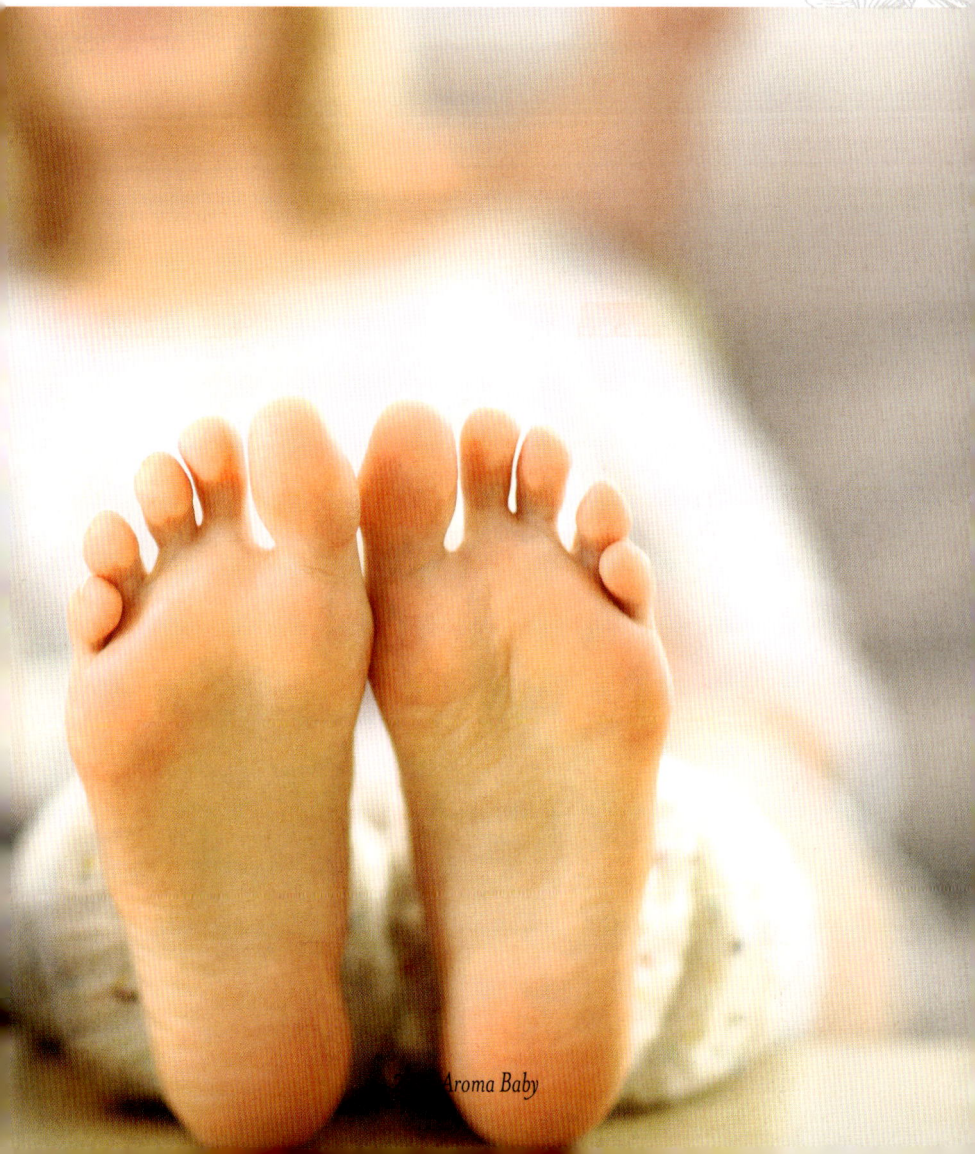

Aroma Baby

Start by pressing firmly and then releasing. Avoid applying pressure to any particular pressure point too long. You may continue along the acupressure points and meridians or use the reflexology or Vita Flex points as well. Once you have completed small point stimulations, massage the general area with the essential oil.

Warm Compress

For deeper penetration, use a warm compress after applying essential oils. Completely soak the cloth or towel by placing it in comfortably hot water. By the time you wring out the cloth and shake it, it will be a nice, warm temperature to be placed on the location. Then, cover the cloth loosely with a dry towel or blanket to seal in the heat. Leave the cloth on for 15-30 minutes. Remove the cloth immediately if there is any discomfort.

Cold Packs

Apply essential oils on the location, followed by cold water or ice packs when treating inflamed or swollen tissues. Frozen packages of peas or corn make excellent ice packs that will mold to the contours of the body part. Keep the cold pack on until the swelling diminishes.

For neurological problems, always use cold packs, never hot ones.

Layering

This technique consists of applying multiple oils one at a time. For example, rub Marjoram over a sore muscle, massage it into the tissue gently until the area is dry, and then apply a second oil such as Peppermint until the oil is absorbed and the skin is dry. Then layer on the third oil, such as Basil, and continue massaging.

Making a Compress

- Rub 1–3 drops on the location, diluted or neat, depending on the oil used and the skin sensitivity at that location.
- Cover the location with a hot, damp towel.
- Cover the moist towel with a dry towel for 10–30 minutes, depending on individual need.

As the oil penetrates the skin, you may experience a warming or even a burning sensation, especially in areas where the greatest benefits occur. If burning becomes uncomfortable, apply V-6 Vegetable Oil Complex, a massage oil, or any pure vegetable oil such as olive, coconut, or almond to the location.

A second type of application is very mild and is suitable for children or those with sensitive skin.

- Place 5-15 drops of essential oil into a basin filled with warm water.
- Water temperature should be approximately 100° F (38° C), unless the patient suffers neurological conditions; in that case, use cool water.
- Vigorously agitate the water and let it stand for 1 minute.
- Place a dry face cloth on top of the water to soak up oils that have floated to the surface.
- Wring out the water and apply the cloth on the location. To seal in the warmth, cover the location with a thick towel for 15–30 minutes.

Bath

Adding essential oils to bath water is challenging because oil does not mix with water. For even dispersion, mix 5–10 drops of essential oil in 1/4 cup of Epsom salts or bath gel base and then put the cup under a running faucet and gradually add water. This method will help the oils disperse in the bath evenly and prevent stronger oils from stinging sensitive areas.

You can also use premixed bath gels and shampoos containing essential oils as a liquid soap in the shower or bath. Lather down with the bath gel, let it soak in, and then rinse. To maximize benefits, leave the soap or shampoo on the skin or scalp for several minutes to allow the essential oils to penetrate.

You can create your own aromatic bath gels by placing 5–15 drops of essential oil in 1/2 oz. of an unscented bath gel base and then add to the bath water as described above.

Shower

Essential oils can be added to Epsom salts and used in the shower. There are special shower heads containing an attached receptacle that can be filled with the essential oil/salts mixture. This allows essential oils to not only make contact with the skin but also diffuses the fragrance of the oils into the air. The shower head receptacle can hold approximately 1/4 to 1/2 cup of bath salts.

Start by adding 5–10 drops of essential oil to 1/4 cup of bath salt. Fill the shower head receptacle with the oil/salt mixture. Make sure neither oils nor salts come in contact with the plastic seal on top of the receptacle. This should provide enough salt material for about 2–3 showers. Some shower heads have a bypass feature that allows the user to switch from aromatic salt water to regular tap water.

How to Enhance the Benefits of Topical Application

The longer essential oils stay in contact with the skin, the more likely they are to be absorbed. You may layer your favorite cream on top of the essential oils to reduce evaporation of the oils and enhance penetration. This may also help seal and protect cuts and wounds.

Do not use ointments on burns until they are at least three days old; however, LavaDerm™ Cooling Mist spray may be used immediately to provide comforting relief for minor burns, abrasions, dryness, and other skin irritations.

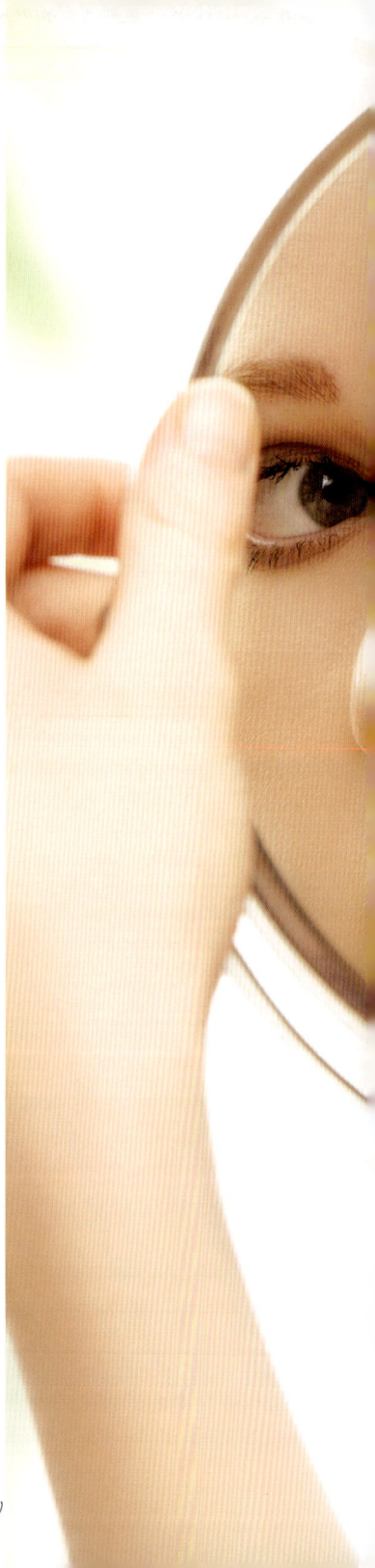

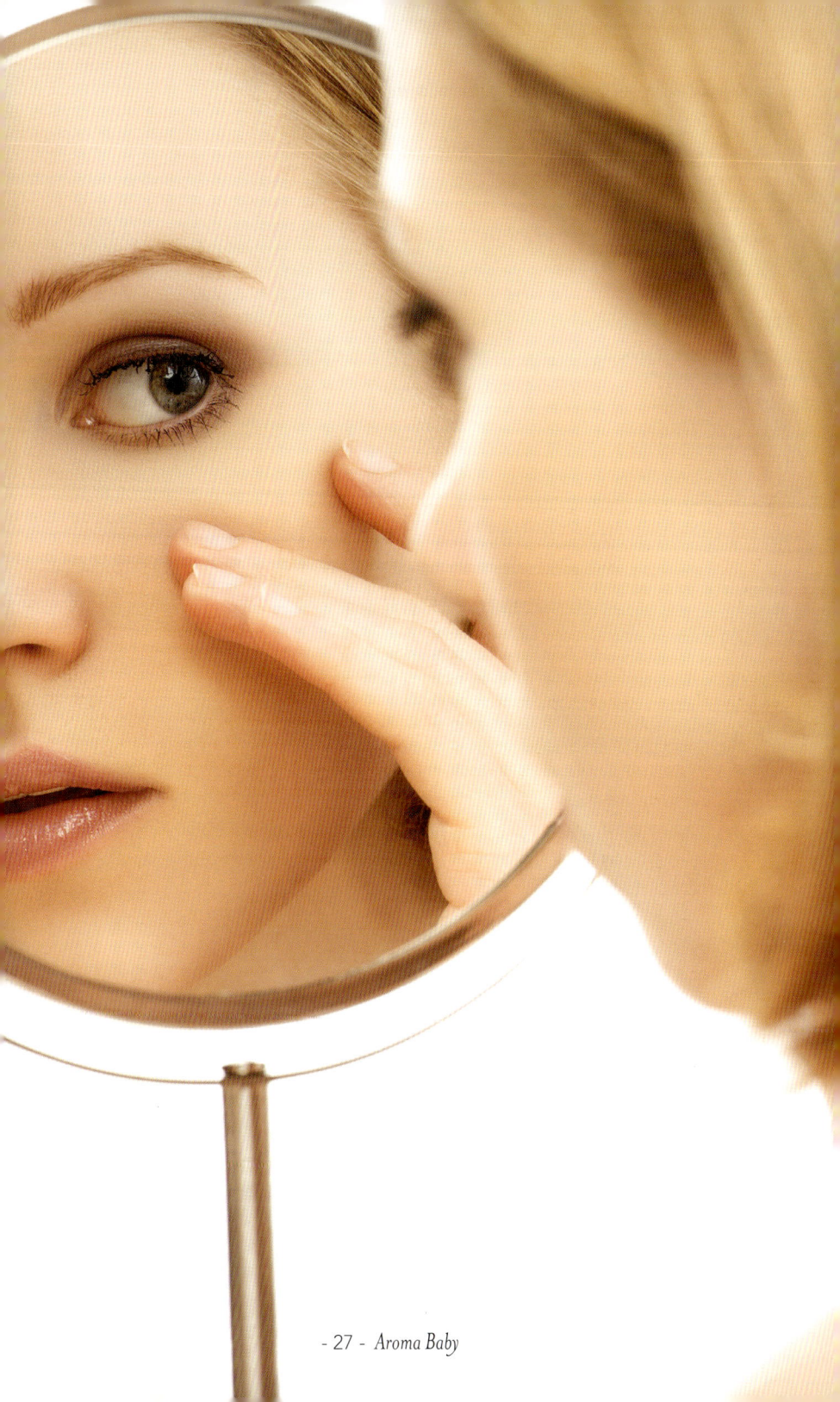

DIFFUSING

Diffused oils alter the structure of molecules that create odors, rather than just masking them. They also increase oxygen availability, produce negative ions, and release natural ozone. Many essential oils such as Lemongrass, Orange, Grapefruit, Tea Tree (Melaleuca Alternifolia), Eucalyptus Globulus, Lavender, Frankincense, and Lemon, along with essential oil blends (Purification, Melrose, and Thieves), are extremely effective for eliminating and destroying airborne germs and bacteria.

A cold-air diffuser is designed to atomize a microfine mist of essential oils into the air, where they can remain suspended for several hours. Unlike aroma lamps or candles, a diffuser disperses essential oils without heating or burning, which can render the oil therapeutically less beneficial and even create toxic compounds. Research shows that cold-air diffusing certain oils may:

- Reduce bacteria, fungus, mold, and unpleasant odors
- Relax the body, relieve tension, and clear the mind
- Help with weight management
- Improve concentration, alertness, and mental clarity
- Stimulate neurotransmitters
- Stimulate secretion of endorphins
- Stimulate growth hormone production and receptivity
- Improve the secretion of IgA antibodies that fight candida
- Improve digestive function
- Improve hormonal balance
- Relieve headaches

Guidelines for Diffusing

- Check the viscosity or thickness of the oil you want to diffuse. If the oil has too much natural wax and is too thick, it could plug the diffuser and make cleaning difficult.
- Start by diffusing oils for 15–30 minutes a day. As you become accustomed to the oils and recognize their effects, you may increase the diffusing time to 1–2 hours per day.
- By connecting your diffuser to a timer, you can gain better control over the length and duration of diffusing. For some respiratory conditions, you may diffuse the oils the entire night.

- Do not use more than one blend at a time in a diffuser, as this may alter the smell and the therapeutic benefit. However, a single oil may be added to a blend when diffusing.
- Place the diffuser high in the room so that the oil mist falls through the air and removes the odor-causing substances.
- If you want to wash the diffuser before using a different oil blend, use Thieves Household Cleaner with warm water or any natural soap and warm water.
- If you do not have a diffuser, you can add several drops of essential oil to a spray bottle with 1 cup purified water and shake. You can use this to mist your entire house, workplace, or car.

Other Ways to Diffuse Oils

- Add your favorite essential oils to cedar chips to make your own potpourri.
- Put scented cedar chips in your closets or drawers to deodorize them.
- Put essential oils on cotton balls or tissues and place them in your car, home, work, or hotel heating or air conditioning vents.
- Put a few drops of oil in a bowl or pan of water and set it on a warm stove.
- On a damp cloth, sprinkle a few drops of one of your purifying essential oils and place the cloth near an intake duct of your heating and cooling system so that the air can carry the aroma throughout your home.

OTHER USES

Direct Inhalation:

- Place 2 or more drops into the palm of your left hand and rub clockwise with the flat palm of your right hand. Cup your hands together over your nose and mouth and inhale deeply. (Do not touch your eyes!)
- Add several drops of an essential oil to a bowl of hot (not boiling) water. Inhale the steaming vapors that rise from the bowl. To increase the intensity of the oil vapors inhaled, drape a towel over your head and the bowl before inhaling.

- Apply oils to a cotton ball or tissue (do not use synthetic fibers or fabric) and place it in the air vent of your car.
- Inhale directly.

Indirect or Subtle Inhalation:
(Wearing as a perfume or cologne)
- Rub 2 or more drops of oil on your chest, neck, upper sternum, wrists, or under your nose and ears, and enjoy the fragrance throughout the day.
- Diffusion

VITA FLEX TECHNIQUE

Vita Flex means "vitality through the reflexes" and is an easy way to apply essential oils through the bottoms of the feet. It is a very important technique that can facilitate the relief of pain and suffering quickly as well as improving physical and emotional well-being.

During pregnancy, the feet may be one of the best places to apply essential oils. In the first two trimesters, you can most likely apply the oils yourself. As you progress into your third trimester, you may need someone to help you.

Vita Flex is a specialized form of hand and foot massage that is exceptionally effective in delivering the benefits of essential oils throughout the body. The technique is based on a complete network of reflex points that stimulate all the internal body systems. When the fingertips connect to specific reflex

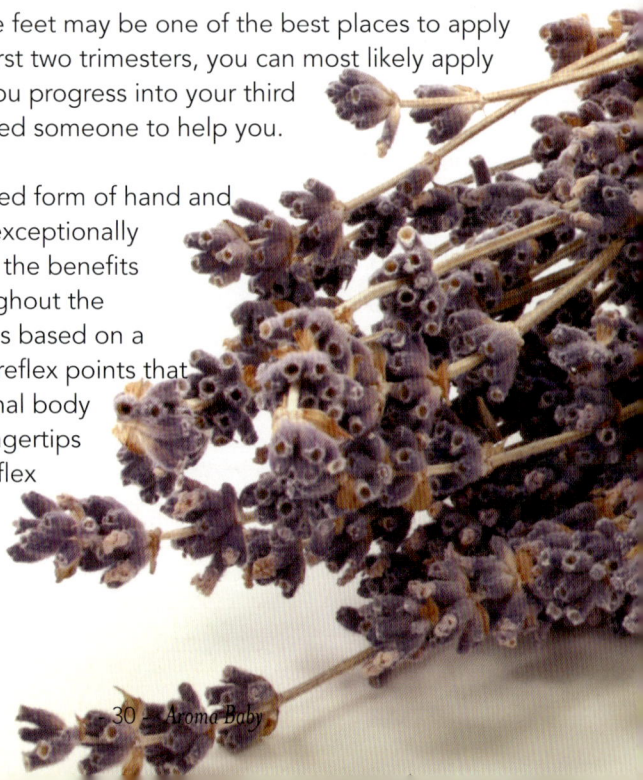

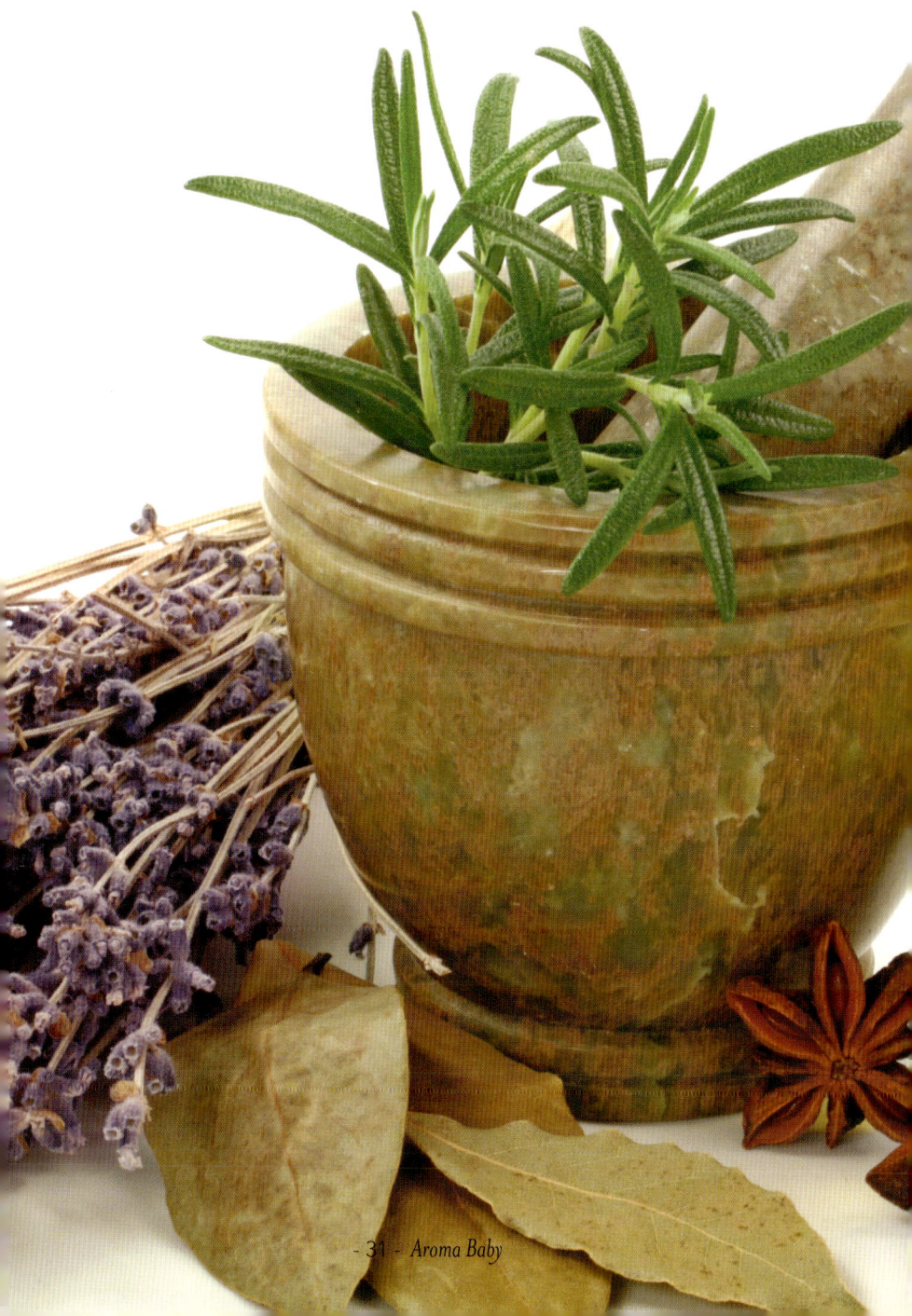

points with essential oils using the special Vita Flex application, an electrical charge is released that sends energy through the neuroelectrical pathways. This electrical charge follows the pathways of the nervous system to where there is a break in the electrical circuit, usually related to an energy block caused by toxins, damaged tissues, or loss of oxygen.

Vita Flex helps to correct weakened or injured areas through the electrical reflex points, preventing further injury, lessening stress and allowing for quicker, more efficient healing. Combining the electrical frequency of the oils and that of the person receiving the application creates rapid and phenomenal results.

This ancient technique offers you an additional way to care for your health during pregnancy.

Vita Flex on the Hands

The hands also have specific reflex points that correspond to different organs and systems of the body. Although the hands are smaller and perhaps not as comfortable to work on, if you are in a hurry or are unable to get to the feet, there are still definite benefits in using the Vita Flex technique on the hands.

RAINDROP TECHNIQUE

In the case of Raindrop Technique, many women find that having a Raindrop massage during pregnancy several times a week helps them stay balanced, manage pain, and have a better outcome. The key is to work with someone who is properly trained and knows how to read your body's cues as they apply the technique.

Skin Warming or Reddening

In the case of Raindrop Technique, the use of certain undiluted essential oils typically causes minor reddening and "heat" in the tissues. Normally, this is perfectly safe and not something to be overly concerned about. Individuals who have fair skin such as blondes and redheads or women whose systems are toxic are more susceptible to this temporary reddening.

Should the reddening or heat become excessive, it can be remedied within a minute or two by immediately applying several drops of V-6 Vegetable Oil Complex or a pure, high quality vegetable oil like jojoba, almond, or coconut oil on the affected area. This effectively dilutes the oils and the warming effect.

Temporary, mild warming is normal for Raindrop Technique. Typically, it is even milder than that of many capsicum creams or sports ointments. Indeed, rather than being a cause of concern, this warming indicates that positive benefits are being received.

In cases where the warmth or heat exceeds your comfort zone, as mentioned before, the facilitator can apply any pure vegetable oil to the area until your comfort level returns to normal and reddening dissipates (usually within 2-5 minutes).

Note: If a rash should appear, it is an indication of a chemical reaction between the oils and synthetic compounds in the skin cells and the interstitial fluid of the body (usually from conventional personal care products).

Some misconstrue this as an allergic reaction, when in fact the problem is not caused by an allergy but rather by foreign chemicals already imbedded in the tissues. Essential oils are known to digest chemicals and other unwanted toxins in the body, and sometimes that process starts to work very quickly.

Medical Professionals

A number of medical professionals throughout the United States have adopted Raindrop Technique in their clinical practice and have found it to be an outstanding method to relieve the problems associated with sciatica, scoliosis, kyphosis, and chronic back pain. Many of these are issues women face during pregnancy.

Mental and Emotional Support

Today we live in a society of emotional turmoil. More and more evidence is accumulating that our emotional health can have a profound effect on our physical health. More than ever before, researchers are probing the impact that emotional states have on the physical condition of the body.

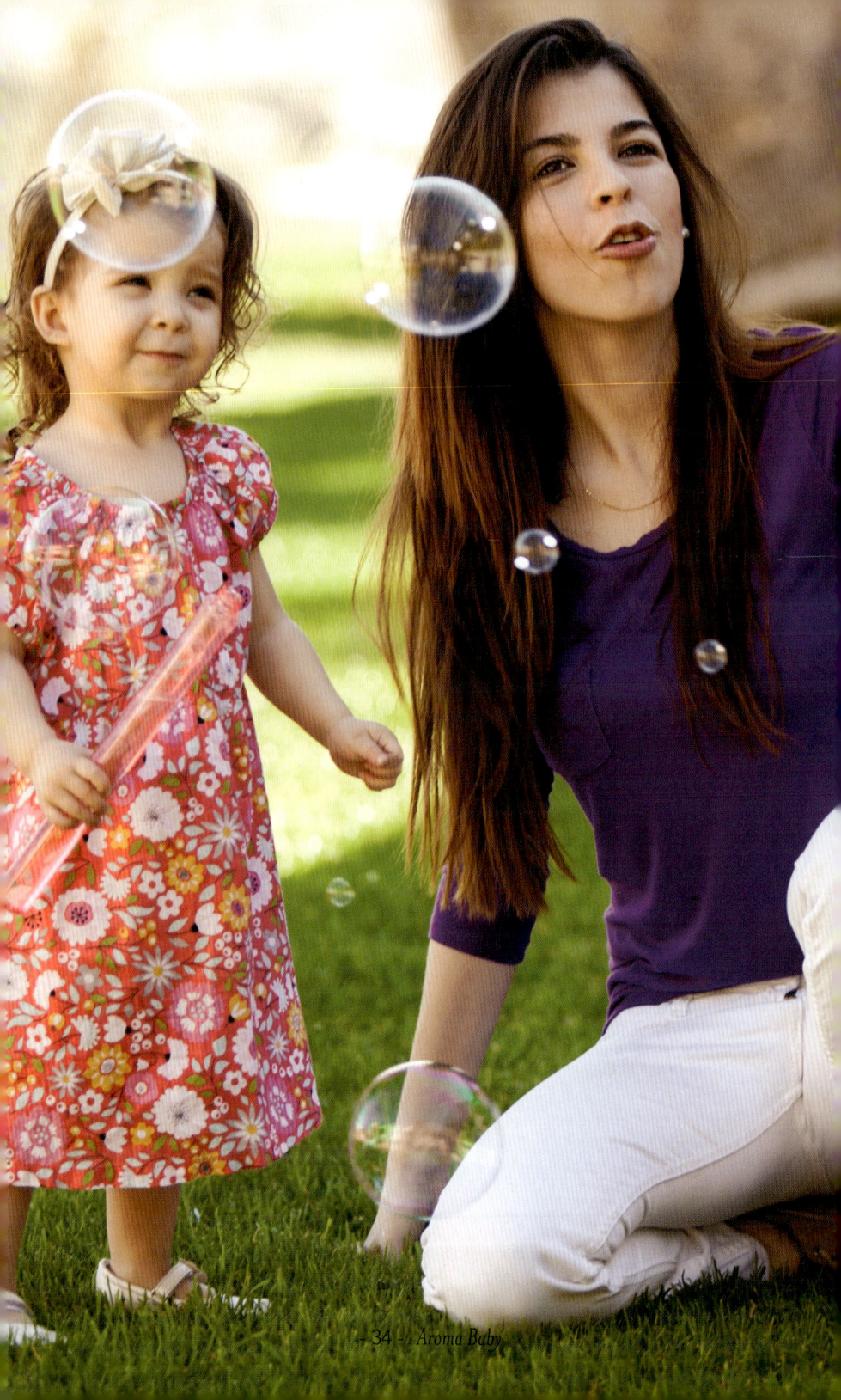

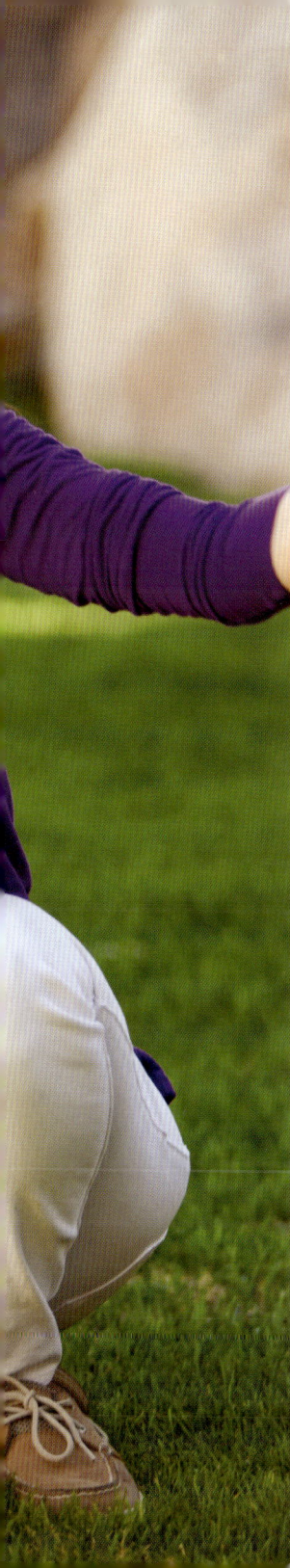

Many doctors are recognizing the possibility that a number of diseases are caused by emotional problems that link back to infancy and childhood—and perhaps even to the womb. These emotional problems can compromise body systems and even genetic structuring through a process that creates the equivalent of a molecular "memory" in key organs and structures of the body.

Emotion and Memory

As scientists have studied to understand the neural basis of emotion, they have discovered that the limbic system of the brain plays a vital role in interpreting and channeling intense experiences, particularly memories of fear or trauma. Interestingly, the two parts of the limbic system that play a major role in emotional processing—the amygdala and the hippocampus—are located within less than an inch of the olfactory nerve.

Olfaction or smell is the sense that is physically the closest to the limbic system structures of the amygdala, which is involved in experiencing emotion and also in emotional memory, and the hippocampus, which encompasses memory: working memory and short-term memory. This gives you an idea of how closely linked the sense of smell is to emotion and memory.

Fear and trauma can produce conditioned emotional responses that—unless released—will not only hamper our ability to live and enjoy life fully but can also limit the ability of some body systems to function properly, particularly the immune system. This can result in unexplained pain and illness as well as depression and other psychological "issues."

Many of the biochemicals in essential oils—particularly sesquiterpenes—can increase blood oxygen levels in the brain. The stimulation of both aroma and oxygenation seems to affect the amygdala in ways that facilitate the release of stored emotional blocks, both in the subconscious and in various body systems.

Combining the aroma of essential oils and oxygenation regularly over time—accompanied by mental focus and intent—has proven to be effective in many cases for resolving unexplained physical problems that were rooted in past emotional trauma.

Relaxing with Essential Oils

Another way in which essential oils can assist in helping people to move beyond emotional blocks is through their relaxing effect. The aldehydes and esters of certain essential oils such as Lavender, RutaVala, Frankincense, etc., are very calming and sedating to the nervous system (including both the sympathetic and parasympathetic systems). These substances allow us to relax instead of getting caught in an anxiety spiral.

Releasing with Essential Oils

The process of emotional release using essential oils should not be dramatic, but gentle, occurring step-by-step over a period of time. Application of the oils accompanied by mental focus and relaxation should occur multiple times per day. Some emotional blocks will require only a day or two to begin releasing; others may require weeks.

BABIES AND CHILDREN

Babies and children respond very well to essential oils and nutritional supplements. The only difference is the amount. Mightyzyme, MightyVites, and NingXia Red are products specific to children. The Super C Chewables are a good companion to MightyVites and Mightyzyme.

Children have an innate sense about essential oils. Most children are very drawn to the aromas. They love to have them massaged on their feet and backs as much as they love to feel them in their own hands and massage them on someone else. They often want to put them on without question or concern.

- **Babies:** Put 1–2 drops of oil in your hand and rub your hands together until they are practically dry. Then hold them over any area of the baby. This works very well without direct application.
- **Direct application:** Mix 1–2 drops of an essential oil in V-6 Vegetable Oil Complex and apply to the bottoms of feet.
- **Children:** Put 1–2 drops on bottoms of feet or anywhere else on the body as long as the oil is diluted in V-6 Vegetable Oil Complex or in any vegetable oil. Although dilution is recommended, it is not always necessary. The essential oil roll-ons are perfect for babies and children of all ages as well as for adults.

Fortifying the Immune System

Nothing will help you in your pregnancy like a strong immune system. You have not only to protect yourself from disease, but also impart immune support to your baby. The immune system must be strong and responsive in order to combat all types of disease brought on by pollution and undigested toxins that can lower the immune system response. Dietary supplements containing essential oils can boost and strengthen the immune system. The following supplements are infused by a balance of essential oils and other active ingredients:

ImmuPro™—combines complex polysaccharides, beta glucans, minerals, essential oils, and melatonin, one of the most powerful immune stimulants known.
- Take 1 or more chewable tablets at night before retiring. Some people enjoy the taste as well as the added benefits of 3–4 tablets. If you take them during the day, you will probably feel like you would like to take a nap.

  Children love them and so do parents who have a hard time getting their children to sleep. Try ½ tablet to begin with, and that may be sufficient. However, 1–2 tablets are not harmful and may even be "helpful."

Sulfurzyme®—contains MSM and NingXia wolfberry for powerful nutritional support.
- Maintenance: 1–2 teaspoons daily in water or juice or as needed
- Additional health support: Begin with 1–2 teaspoons daily and work up to 3–4 tablespoons daily or more if desired

ImmuPower™—is an essential oil blend used to strengthen, build, and protect the body.
- Maintenance: 1 capsule 3–4 times weekly
- Pneumonia, flu, or colds: 4 capsules daily for 10 days, rest 4 days, and then 1 capsule daily for another 10 days

Inner Defense™—Take 2–4 capsules daily

OmegaGize3®—Take 1–2 capsules daily

Super B™—Take 1 tablet daily after eating

Thyromin™—is a very unique blend of glandular extracts, herbs, amino acids, minerals, and essential oils to support the thyroid. This gland regulates body metabolism and temperature and is important for immune function.
- Maintenance: Take 1 capsule immediately before going to bed.
- Additional health support: Take 3 capsules immediately before going to bed and 2 in the morning.

Mineral Essence™—is a precisely balanced complex of essential oils and more than 60 trace minerals that are essential to a healthy immune system. It includes well-known antioxidants and immune-supporters such as zinc, selenium, and magnesium.
- Maintenance: Take 1–2 drops 1–3 times daily in water or NingXia Red.
- Additional health support: Take 2–5 drops 2 times daily.

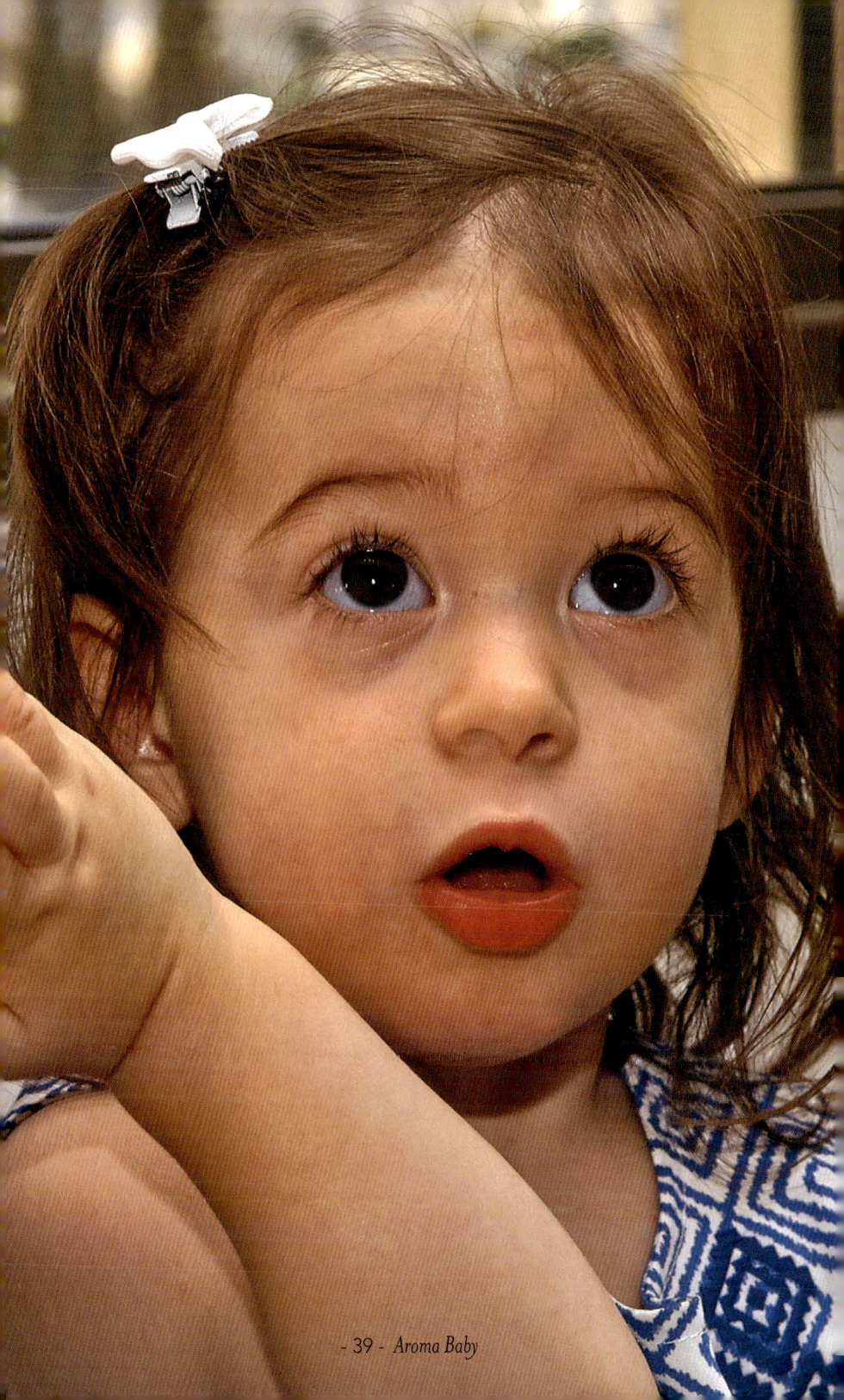

Supplements: Super B™, MultiGreens™, Power Meal™, Pure Protein™, Rehemogen™, AlkaLime™, Ultra Young Plus™, Life 5, NingXia® Red, JuvaTone™, Super C™, and Inner Defense

NingXia Red® Juice is the highest-ranked antioxidant liquid dietary supplement that combines the wolfberry fruit (Lycium barbarum), pomegranates, blueberries, raspberries, and other fruit juices with essential oils. It is delicious and provides a great many nutrients that promote strength, vitality, and longevity.

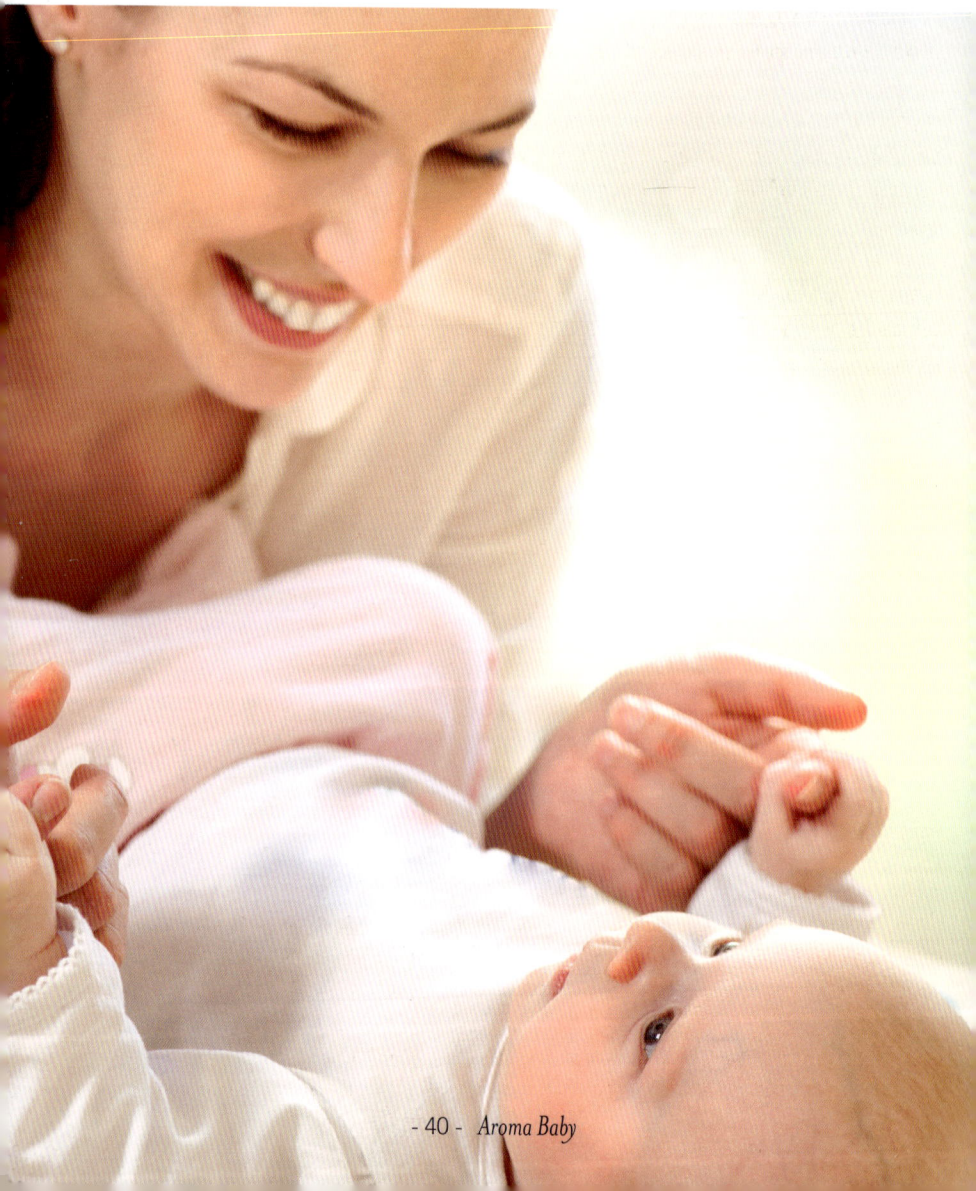

GOOD EATING HABITS

During your pregnancy, you'll encounter many cravings and many foods that sound unappetizing. These foods and preferences may be the complete opposite of what you ordinarily like and dislike. It's important to recognize your cravings but create a healthy balanced diet for you and the baby.

Breakfast is the most important meal of the day. While you may have nausea in the morning, it's important to try and eat something mild to get your blood sugar up to normal after fasting overnight.

If you can, eat breakfast between 6 and 7 a.m. Protein and complex carbohydrate foods are best for energy conversion in the morning. Strawberries or raspberries are the only fruits recommended to eat with cereal.

Plain yogurt or Kefir without sweeteners are good sources of acidophilus and bifida bacteria-cultures essential for proper intestinal flora. Sugar, synthetic sweeteners, and other foods high on the glycemic index should be avoided.

Sometimes people who have health challenges and have digestive systems that do not function properly feel better eating fruit like papaya, mango, pineapple, and watermelon, which are easier to digest.

Cereals can include oatmeal, millet, barley, quinoa, or a mixture of these, with coconut milk, rice milk, almond milk, soy milk, whey powder, or goat milk. However, it is best not to tax the body with too many grains, which make digestion more difficult.

Bread is better toasted to change it from a wet food to a dry food, making it more digestible. However, no bread is healthy for the body if eaten in excess. A and B blood types gain weight more easily than O types because of the difference in digestive systems.

Breakfast is the best time to eat proteins such as beans, rice, eggs, fish, etc., providing more energy and stamina throughout the day. Be sure to take 1–3 Essentialzymes-4 (yellow capsule) with high-protein meals.

Lunch should consist of carbohydrates such as mixed vegetables or salads (particularly greens) along with chicken or turkey, freshwater fish (not farm

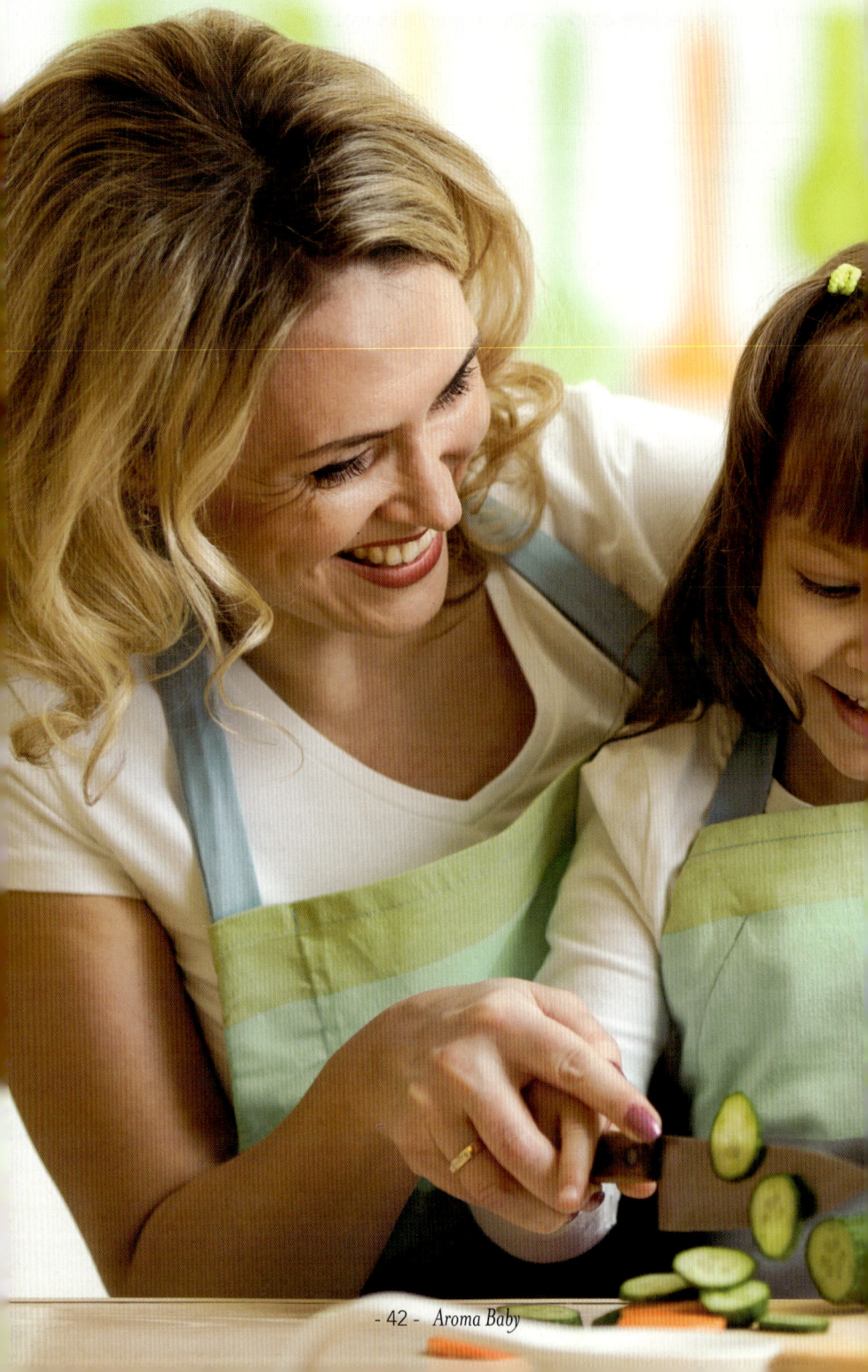

raised), and cage-free chicken. Drink plenty of water with every meal.

A simple meal of organic, white basmati rice with cinnamon, Blue Agave, maple syrup, or Yacon Syrup with coconut milk, almond milk, goat milk, or rice milk is a perfect acid-binding food for an evening meal. White basmati rice is an alkaline food that is easier for the body to digest at night. A Power Meal drink is also a simple replacement meal in the evening.

Dinner should be eaten in the late afternoon or early evening, if possible. It is much better to eat a bigger meal midday and not as heavy in the evening. Both fruit and solid vegetables are suitable for evening meals. If an individual must eat a large, heavy meal late in the day or evening, Essentialzyme or Essentialzymes-4 (yellow capsule) is needed to promote proper digestion, reduce gas, and prevent putrefaction and fungal growth in the intestines.

Healthy Snacks

During pregnancy, most women report a need for snacking. During this time, it's really important to snack in a healthy way. Wolfberry Crisp and Slique Bars are always a treat. They add protein, good fiber, and are packed with nutrients and essential oils that support and strengthen the body.

WATER

Water is imperative during pregnancy because you need to accommodate your body's expansion and the growth of your baby. Nothing is better than clear, cold, spring water. Water is the second most critical substance we need for maintaining life. Without water, life ceases to exist. Water is the activator for all body functions, for growth, development, strength, and vitality. The only substance more important to the body than water is oxygen.

The ideal amount of water to consume is half your body weight in ounces per day. That means if you weigh 160 pounds, you should drink 80 ounces of water or about ten, 8-ounce glasses per day. Lack of water or a state of dehydration may trigger many health conditions such as hypertension, asthma, allergies, migraine headaches, dizziness, and many more.

Because water is so crucial to your life and health and that of your baby, it is crucial that you drink pure water. Choose filtered or purified water that you trust from a dependable source.

BEST PRACTICES

Essential oils are very concentrated, natural substances—easily 100 times more concentrated than the natural herbs and plants from which they are distilled. For this reason it is important to dilute certain essential oils before using them therapeutically.
Other essential oils are so mild that dilution is simply not necessary, even for use on infants.

The five standard methods of application are topical, inhalation, ingestion, oral, and retention. This book focuses mostly on the first four.

Mixing Single Oils and Blends
The essential oil singles and blends listed for a specific condition may be used either separately or together. Combining two single oils, or one single oil with a blend, may often produce a stronger effect than when using them individually.

Usually 1-3 drops of either a single oil or a blend is sufficient, mixing up to 3 or 4 oils in any given combination at a time.

Choosing Your Best Essential Oil to Use

The essential oils you'll find recommended for specific conditions are not the only oils you can use. They are, however, the oils most commonly used with success for those conditions. Other oils not listed can also be effective. Some of this process is trial and error to determine which oils work best for your personal needs and body.

If results are not apparent after trying an oil and waiting a little while, try another single oil, blend, supplement, or combination on the next application. Sometimes you have to keep experimenting until you find what works for you. This is because one particular oil may be more compatible with one person's body chemistry than with another person's chemistry.

Essential oils can be used topically for massage, acupuncture, Raindrop Technique, and Vita Flex on the bottoms of the feet. In most cases, 3-4 drops are sufficient to produce significant effects, unless using a specific protocol.

Most single oils and blends should be diluted 50/50 when putting them on the skin. Oils that definitely should be diluted are oils such as Cistus, Clove, Cypress, Lemongrass, Mountain Savory, Oregano, Rosemary, Thyme, etc. For some people, an oil like Basil might be too "hot" if put neat on the skin; for others, Basil will not be "hot" at all. That is why it is best to always do a skin test before applying any oil. When in doubt, dilute.

When diluting the oils, use the V-6 Vegetable Oil Complex for either topical or internal application, particularly if you have not used essential oils previously. Use no more than 10 to 20 drops during one topical application.

Precautions

When using topically, first do a skin test by putting 1 drop of the desired essential oil on the inside of the upper arm. If cosmetics and personal care products made with synthetic chemicals or soaps and cleansers containing synthetic or petroleum-based chemicals have been used on the skin, then the skin may be uncomfortably sensitive.

If any redness or irritation results, the skin should be thoroughly cleansed; then the oil may be reapplied. If skin irritation persists, try using a different oil or oil blend.

You may want to consider starting an internal cleansing program for 30 days before using essential oils. Use ICP™, ComforTone®, JuvaPower®, Essentialzyme, Detoxzyme®, and other cleansing supplements.

Internal Use

Many essential oils are taken internally as dietary supplements. The Vitality™ line is perfectly labeled for internal use. Try to choose these oils when oral or internal use is suggested. When an oil such as Lemon is listed with Lemon Vitality, the regular oil is best for topical or inhalation while the Vitality oil is best for oral/ingestion.

Some people put 1-3 drops in water to drink, but others use cold NingXia Red or another juice of their choice.

If you prefer to swallow a capsule, you can fill a "00" capsule with oil using an eyedropper. Fill with the number of drops desired and the rest of the capsule with V-6 Vegetable Oil Complex or any other organic vegetable oil. If you are uncertain, consult with someone who is experienced in taking oils internally.

Always drink more water when using essential oils because they can accelerate the detoxification process in the body. If you are not taking in adequate fluids, the toxins could recirculate, causing nausea, headaches, etc.

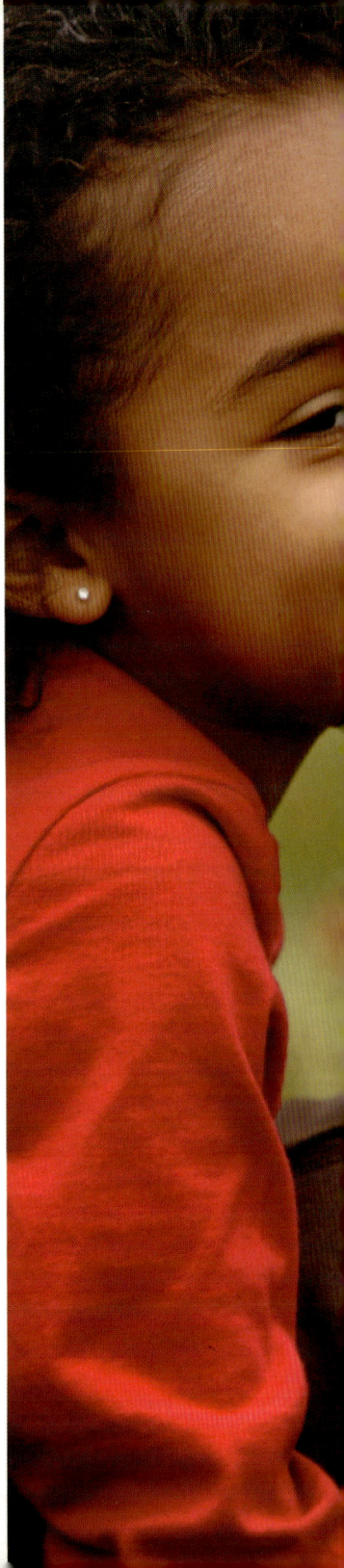

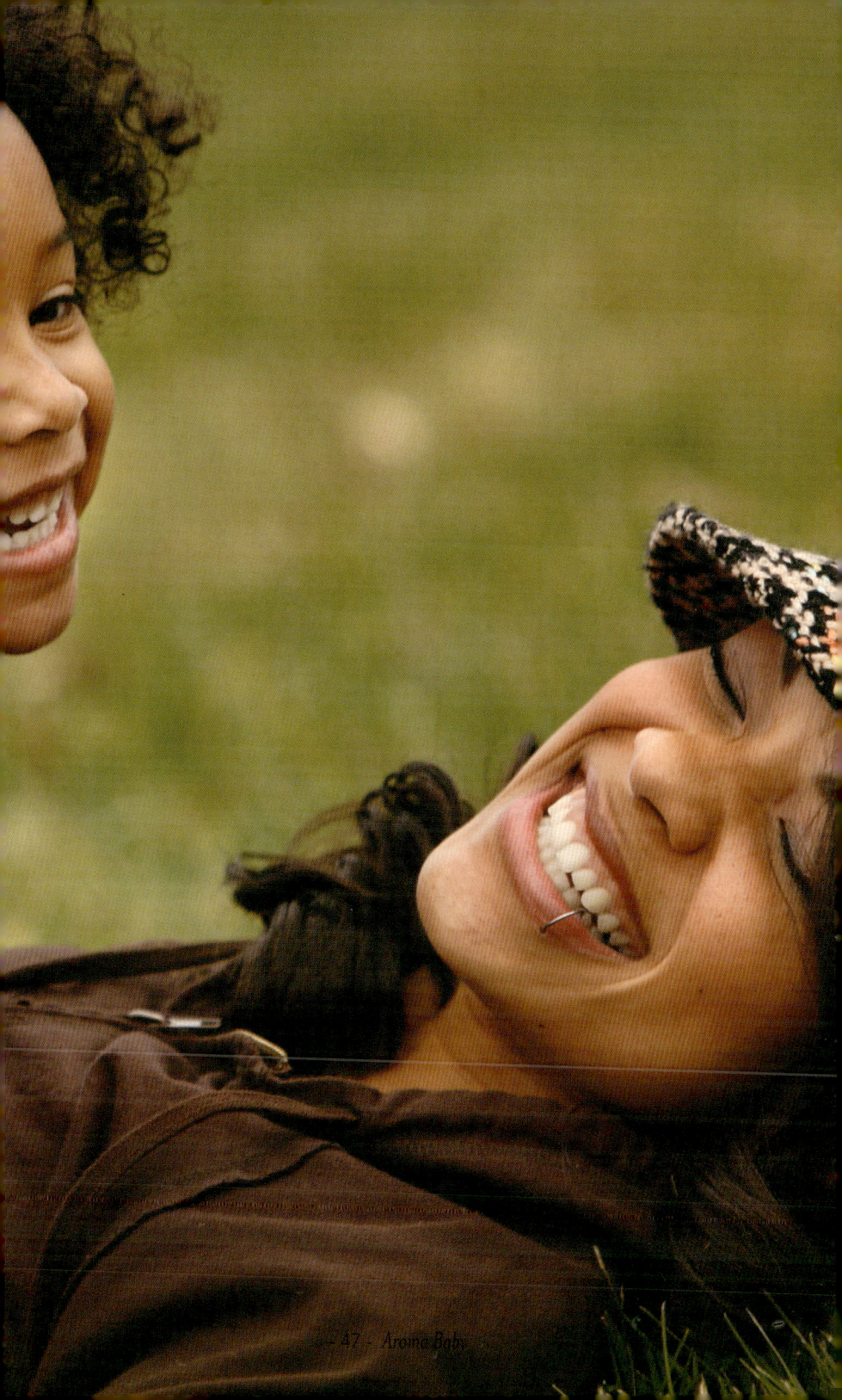

Notes

Notes

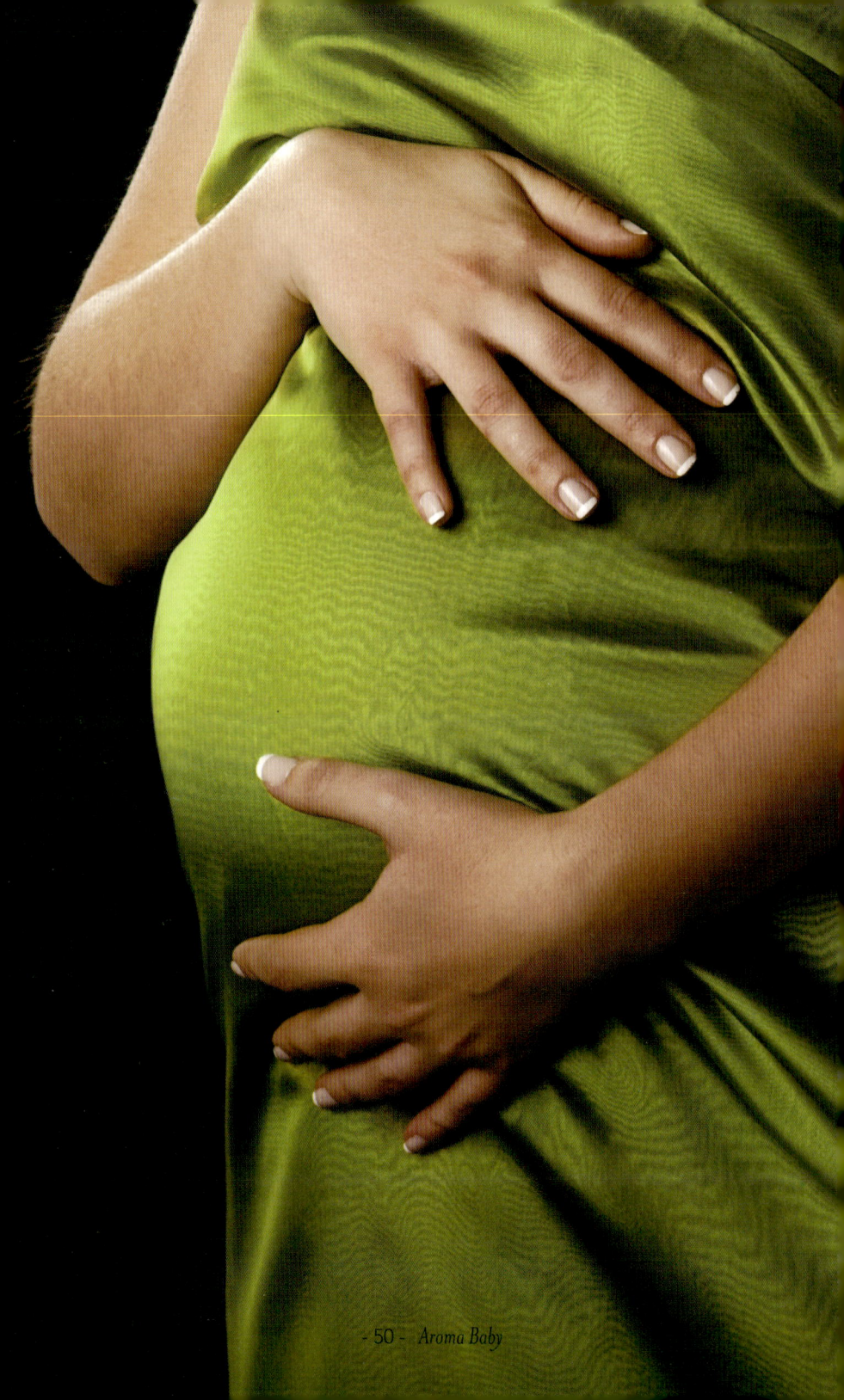

CONDITIONS: MOMS

This section provides recommendations for expecting moms. The solutions include essential oils as well as essential-oil-infused supplemental products. Many of the conditions are common with a normal pregnancy and childbirth. However, always discuss mild to serious conditions with your trusted medical professional. What may begin as a mild condition may be the symptom of something bigger.

ACID REFLUX

Acid reflux can be an unwelcome surprise with pregnancy. It's the backward flow of acid into the esophagus, and it often happens as a result of the hormone changes in pregnancy. These hormones cause the muscles in the esophagus to relax, providing room for the acid to make its way back into the throat. Symptoms can range from acid hiccups and heartburn to pain/burning in the chest.

Recommendations:
AlkaLime
DiGize Vitality
Ginger Vitality
Peppermint Vitality

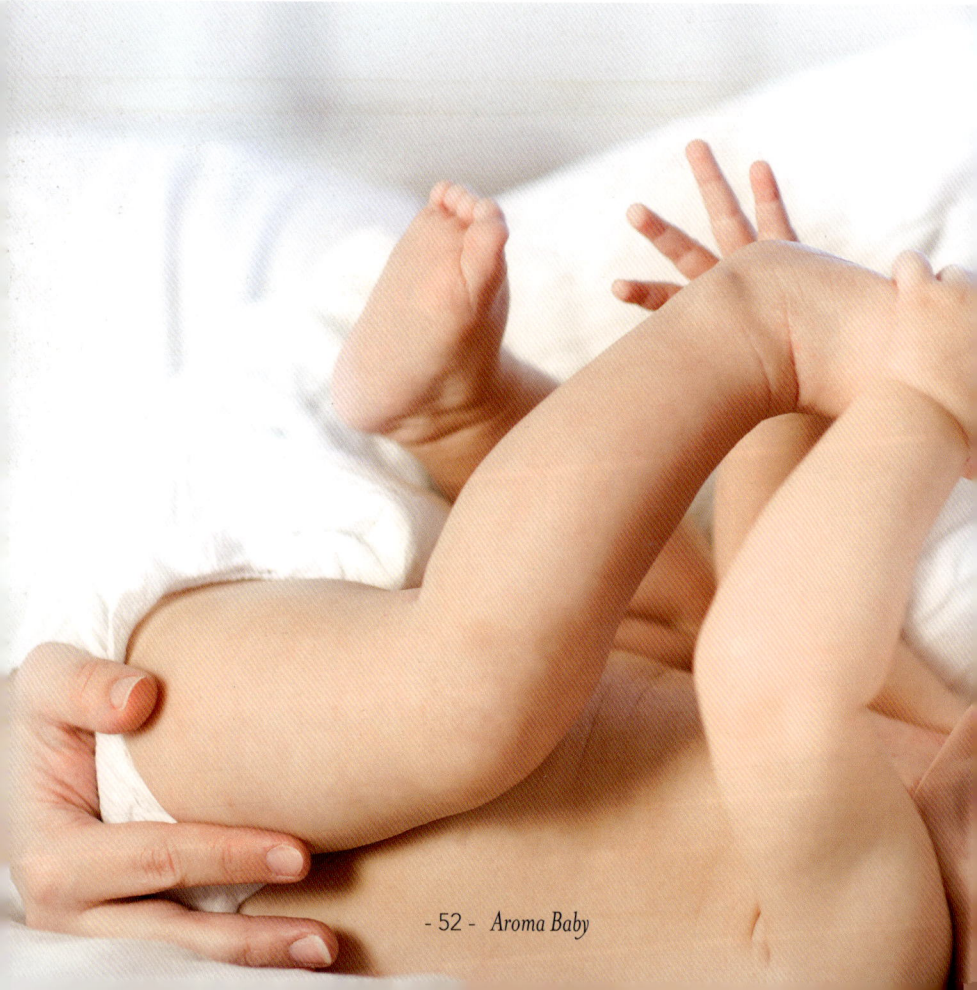

Inhalation:

- Diffuse your choice of oils for ½ hour every 4-6 hours or as desired.
- Put 2-3 drops of your chosen oil in your hands and rub them together, cup your hands over your nose, and inhale throughout the day as needed.
- Put 8-10 drops of oil on a cotton ball or tissue and put it in an air vent in your house, vehicle, hotel room, etc.
- If diffusing while sleeping, set your timer for the desired length of time for automatic shut off.

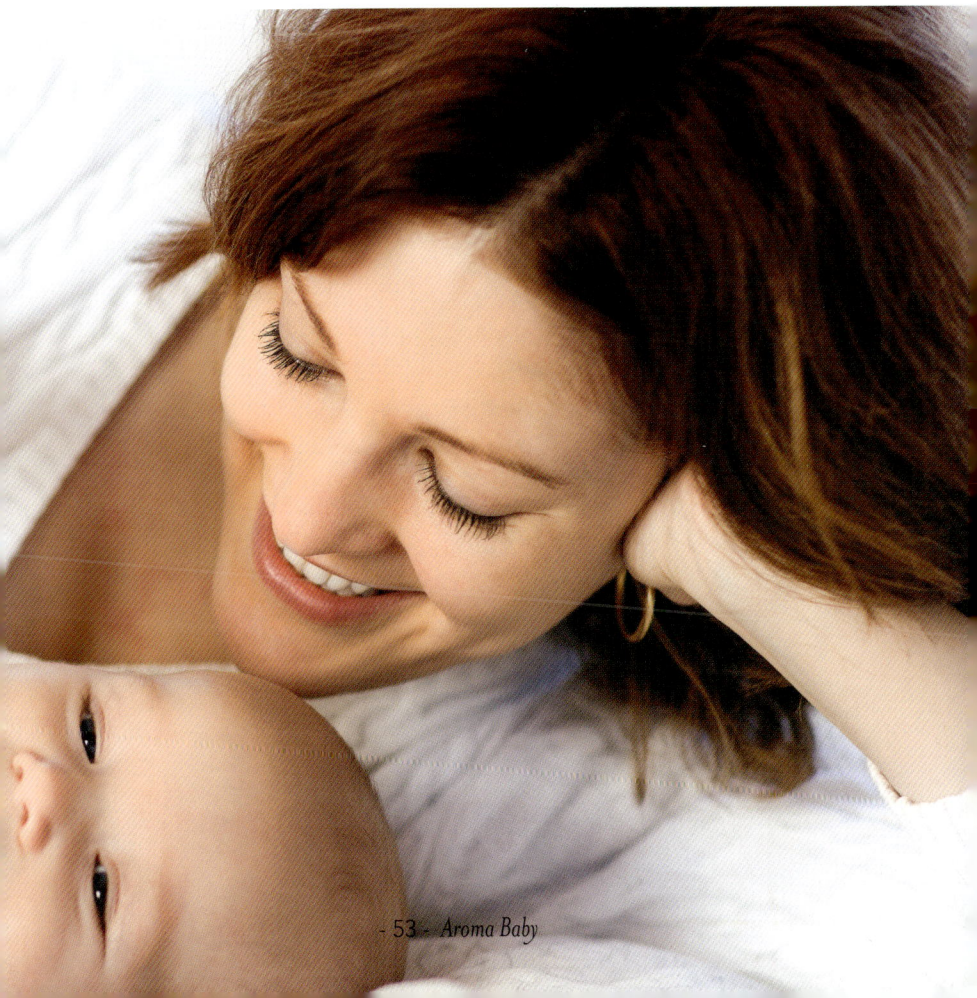

Topical:
- Dilute 50:50 and apply on location 3-6 times daily.
- Place a warm compress with 1-3 drops of recommended oils over stomach.
- Apply recommended oils to the Vita Flex points of the feet.

Ingestion & Oral:
AlkaLime is a safe, effective remedy for acid. Mix one teaspoon in water morning and night to prevent acid. Take after a meal to minimize acid after you've eaten.
- Take 1 capsule with desired Vitality line oil 2 times daily.
- Put 2-3 drops of Vitality line oil in a spoonful of Blue Agave, Yacon Syrup, maple syrup, coconut oil, milk, etc.
- Put the desired amount of oils in a glass of rice milk, almond milk, goat milk, carrot juice, NingXia Red, or even water and then drink it.

ACNE

Just when you thought you were over the teenage acne blues, your pregnancy offers you a second round. Around half of women report acne as a result of pregnancy. Due to the drastic medications on the market that can threaten the wellbeing of your unborn baby, essential oils can be a welcome alternative.

Recommendations:
Bergamot · Claraderm
Frankincense · Geranium
Lavender · Lemon ·
Melrose Orange · Petitgrain
Ravintsara · Rose
Tea Tree
(Melaleuca Alternifolia)

Inhalation:
- Diffuse your choice of oils for ½ hour every 4-6 hours or as desired.
- Put 2-3 drops of your chosen oil in your hands and rub them together, cup your hands over your nose, and inhale throughout the day as needed.
- Put 8-10 drops of oil on a cotton ball or tissue and put it in an air vent in your house, vehicle, hotel room, etc.
- If diffusing while sleeping, set your timer for the desired length of time for automatic shut off.

Topical:

- Apply 4-6 drops diluted 50:50 to forehead, crown of the head, soles of the feet, lower abdomen, and lower back 1-3 times daily.
- Dab 1-2 drops on blemishes twice daily.

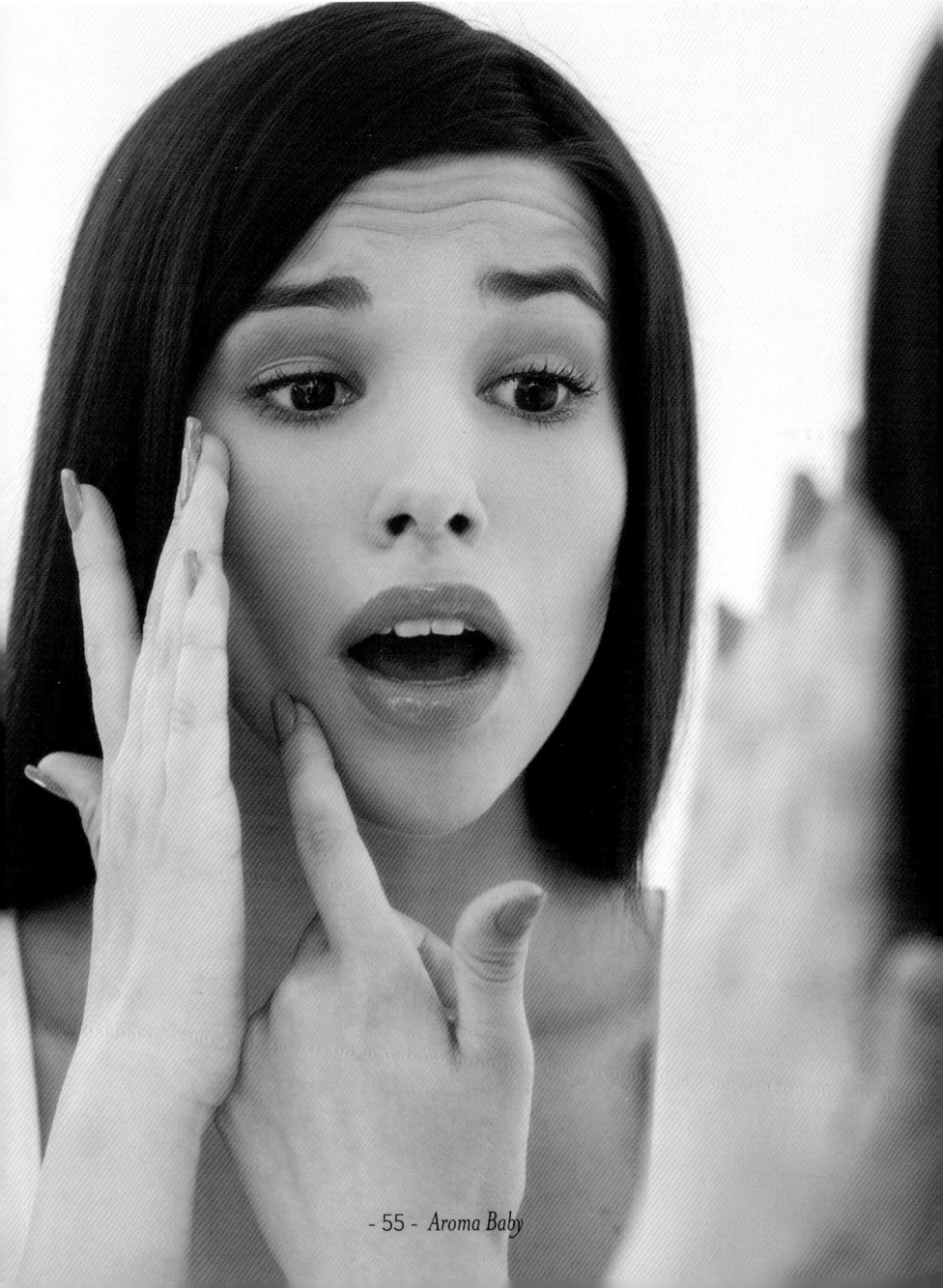

AFTER BIRTH - POSTPARTUM

This is that joyful, exultant—yet exhausting time when moms need special attention for the best recovery. Essential oils can be helpful in multiple ways by lifting mood, boosting energy, and enhancing the healing process.

Recommendations:
ClaraDerm · Frankincense
Gentle Baby · Helichrysum
Joy · Lavender · Melissa
Sacred Frankincense

Inhalation:
- Diffuse recommended oils for 20 minutes 3 times daily.
- Put 2-3 drops of recommended oil in your hands and rub them together, cup your hands over your nose, and inhale 4-6 times daily.
- Put 8-10 drops of oil on a cotton ball or tissue and put it in an air vent in your house, vehicle, hotel room, etc.
- If diffusing while sleeping, set your timer for the desired length of time for automatic shut off.

Topical:
- Apply 2-4 drops neat on temples and back of neck 2-4 times daily or as needed.
- Applying a single drop under the nose is helpful and refreshing.
- Place a warm compress with 1-2 drops of chosen oil on the back.

ASTHMA

Asthmatic moms-to-be can be at higher risk than their non-asthmatic counterparts. It affects 4-8 percent of pregnant women, and keeping it under control will help prevent potentially serious complications.

Recommendations:
Dorado Azul
Eucalyptus Radiata
Sacred Frankincense
Ravintsara · Palo Santo

Inhalation:
- Diffuse your choice of oils for 3-5 minutes or as often as it is comfortable.
- Put 2-3 drops of your chosen oil in your hands and rub them together, cup your hands over your nose, and inhale throughout the day as needed.

- Put 8-10 drops of oil on a cotton ball or tissue and put it in an air vent in your house, vehicle, hotel room, etc.
- If diffusing while sleeping, set your timer for the desired length of time for automatic shut off.

Topical:
- Apply 1-2 drops mixed with Ortho Ease®, Relaxation™, or Sensation™ massage oils on temples and back of neck as desired.
- You may also apply 2-3 drops on the Vita Flex points on the feet and hands.

ATHLETE'S FOOT

There's never a right time for a fungal foot infection, but many women report having one during pregnancy. This may be the result of wearing their most comfortable shoes a little too often or because the hormonal changes make them more susceptible. In either case, several essential oils can provide some relief.

Topical:
- Apply 2-4 drops of oil diluted 50:50 on location 3-5 times daily.

Recommendations:
Melrose
Lavender
Peppermint
Purification
Tea Tree
(Melaleuca Alternifolia)

BACK PAIN

Expecting mothers can be particularly susceptible to back pain during pregnancy and postpartum due to the weight gain, hormone changes, muscle separation, and shift in center of gravity associated with pregnancy.

Topical:
- Apply 2-4 drops neat on specific area 1-3 times daily or as needed.

Recommendations:
AromaSiez™ · Copaiba
Deep Relief™
Deep Relief Roll-On
Idaho Balsam Fir · Marjoram
PanAway™ · Relieve It
Valor™ · Wintergreen

- Apply 2-4 drops on Vita Flex area of foot.
- Use warm compress with 1-2 drops of chosen oil on the back daily.
- Apply Raindrop Technique 2 times weekly for 3 weeks.

For a Back Relief blend, combine:
- 5 drops Wintergreen
- 3 drops Lavender
- 3 drops Idaho Balsam Fir
- 2 drops Marjoram

BATHING

Bath time can be a welcome relief for pregnant mothers, providing they have the proper support getting in and out of the tub to avoid slipping and falling.

Recommendations:
KidScents Bath Gel™
Lavender · Frankincense
Joy · Rose · Ylang Ylang

Topical:
Add desired oil to bath salts or Young Living Bath Base Gel and incorporate into daily bathing.

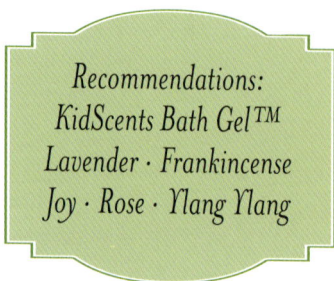

BELCHING

The higher levels of progesterone during pregnancy can slow digestion and lead to gas, bloating, burping, and belching. In the latter part of a pregnancy, the uterus puts pressure on the abdominal cavity, and this has some undesired effects on the digestive tract.

Recommendations:
AlkaLime · DiGize Vitality
Ginger Vitality
Grapefruit Vitality
Peppermint
Peppermint Vitality
Spearmint
Spearmint Vitality

Topical:
- Dilute 50:50 and apply on location 3-6 times daily.
- Place a warm compress with 1-3 drops of recommended oil over the stomach and abdomen.

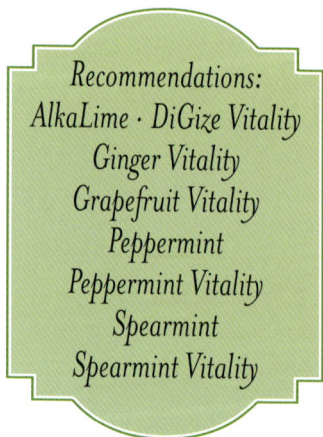

Ingestion & Oral:

- Take 1 capsule with desired Vitality line oil 2 times daily.
- Put 2-3 drops of Vitality line oil in a spoonful of Blue Agave, Yacon Syrup, maple syrup, coconut oil, milk, etc.
- Put the desired amount of oils in a glass of rice milk, almond milk, goat milk, carrot juice, NingXia Red, or even water and then drink it.

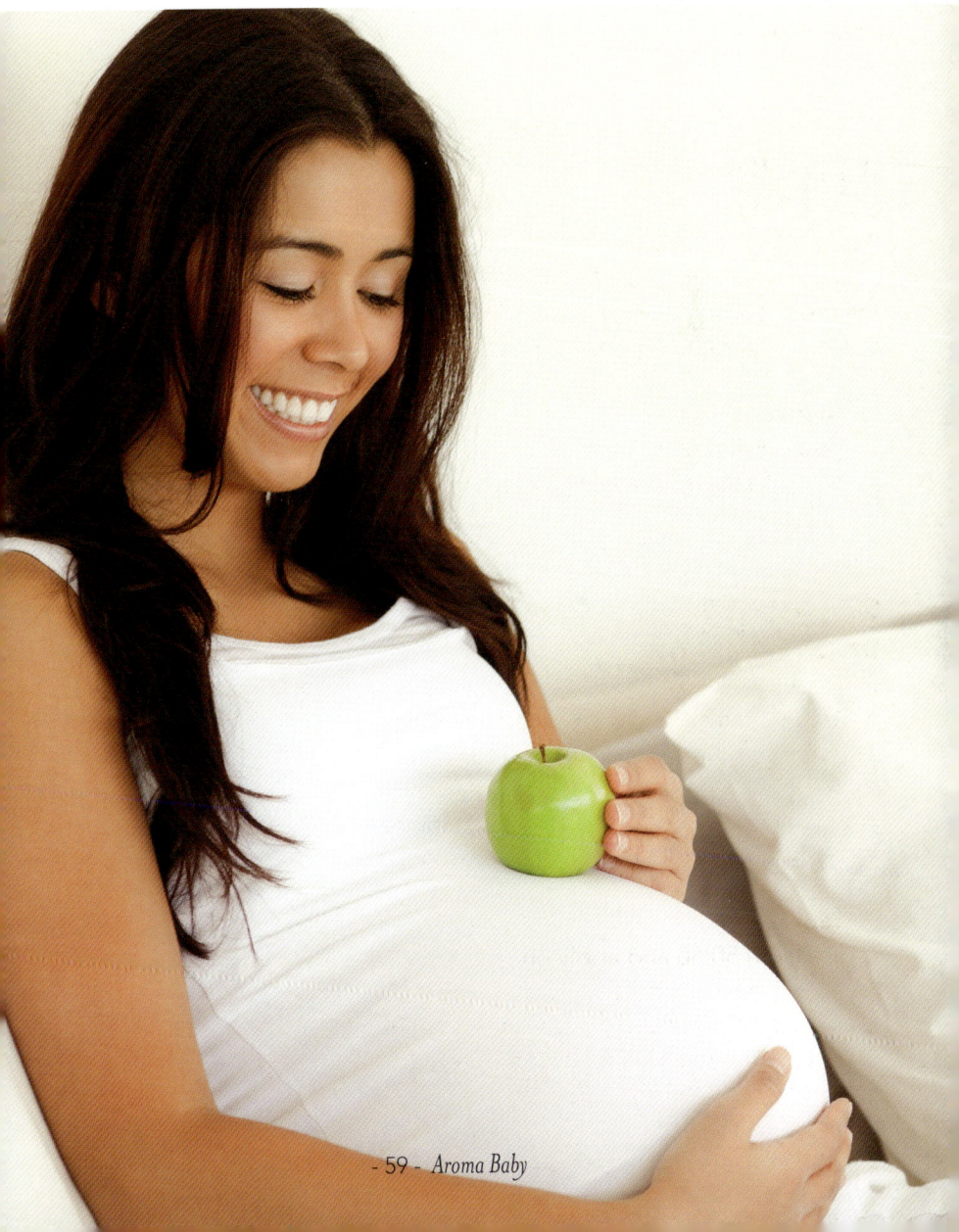

BLADDER

Pregnant women often find themselves going to the bathroom much more frequently than they ordinarily would. This is due to the hormonal changes that cause blood to flow more quickly through the kidneys. Also, the uterus puts some pressure on the bladder, particularly in the latter half of the pregnancy.

Recommendations:
Melrose
Valor
Peace & Calming

Topical:
- Apply 6-8 drops diluted 50:50 on the back over the kidney area as needed.
- Applying a single drop under the nose is helpful and refreshing.
- Massage 2-4 drops of oil neat on the soles of the feet just before bedtime. Children with kidney disorders may especially benefit from this application.
- Place a warm compress with 1-2 drops of chosen oil on the back 1-2 times daily.

BLEEDING

These recommendations are for minor external bleeding only. In the case of vaginal bleeding or passing a stool that would indicate internal bleeding, seek immediate medical attention.

Recommendations:
Cistus · Geranium
Helichrysum · Myrrh
Rose Ointment · Tsuga

Topical: (Wound Compress Blend)
- 5 drops Geranium
- 5 drops Lemon
- 5 drops German Chamomile
- 2 drops Helichrysum

Application:
- Apply 1-2 drops neat (undiluted) on the location of small wounds.
- You may also apply 2-3 drops on the Vita Flex points of the feet.
- Place a cold compress diluted with 1-2 drops of Wound Compress Blend, Helichrysum, Myrrh, etc.

BLOATING

This is often the result of natural slowing of the digestive tract during pregnancy and pressure from the uterus exerted on the abdominal cavity.

Recommendations:
DiGize
DiGize Vitality
Peppermint
Peppermint Vitality

Topical:
- Apply 6-10 drops neat or diluted 50:50 on stomach area as desired.
- Applying a single drop under the nose is helpful and refreshing.
- Place a warm compress with 1-3 drops of recommended oil over the stomach area and Vita Flex points of the feet.

Ingestion & Oral:
- Take 1 capsule with desired Vitality line oil 2 times daily.
- Put 2-3 drops of Vitality line oil in a spoonful of Blue Agave, Yacon Syrup, maple syrup, coconut oil, milk, etc.
- Put the desired amount of oils in a glass of rice milk, almond milk, goat milk, carrot juice, NingXia Red, or even water and then drink it.

BLOOD PRESSURE

Hypertension (high blood pressure above 140/90) can be a serious threat to pregnancy and result in dire complications. If high blood pressure continues after 20 weeks, it can develop into preeclampsia. Many medications can cause problems in pregnant women, so essential oils may provide a safe and natural alternative. Always consult your medical professional if you suspect or know you have high blood pressure during pregnancy.

Recommendations:
Aroma Life™
Bergamot · Clary Sage
Frankincense · Jasmine
Lavender · NingXia Red
Ylang Ylang

Inhalation:
- Diffuse your choice of oils for ½ hour 3 times daily.
- Inhalation of Jasmine reduces anxiety in some people and may help to lower blood pressure.

- Put 2-3 drops of your chosen oil in your hands and rub them together, cup your hands over your nose, and inhale throughout the day as needed.
- Put 8-10 drops of oil on a cotton ball or tissue and put it in an air vent in your house, vehicle, hotel room, etc.
- If diffusing while sleeping, set your timer for the desired length of time for automatic shut off.

Topical:
- Apply 1-3 drops oil diluted 20:80 for a full body massage daily.
- Rub 1-2 drops of oil on the temples and back of neck several times daily.
- Place a warm compress with 1-2 drops of chosen oil on the back.
- For 3 minutes, massage 1-2 drops each of Aroma Life and Ylang Ylang (or Amazonian Ylang Ylang) on the heart Vita Flex point and over the heart and carotid arteries along the neck.
- Notice how the blood pressure will begin to drop within 5-20 minutes. Monitor the pressure and reapply as desired.

Ingestion & Oral:
- NingXia Red can be a great help for stabilizing blood pressure, particularly when taken regularly.
- Consider increasing your intake of magnesium, which acts as a smooth-muscle relaxant and as a natural calcium channel blocker for the heart, lowering blood pressure and dilating the heart blood vessels.

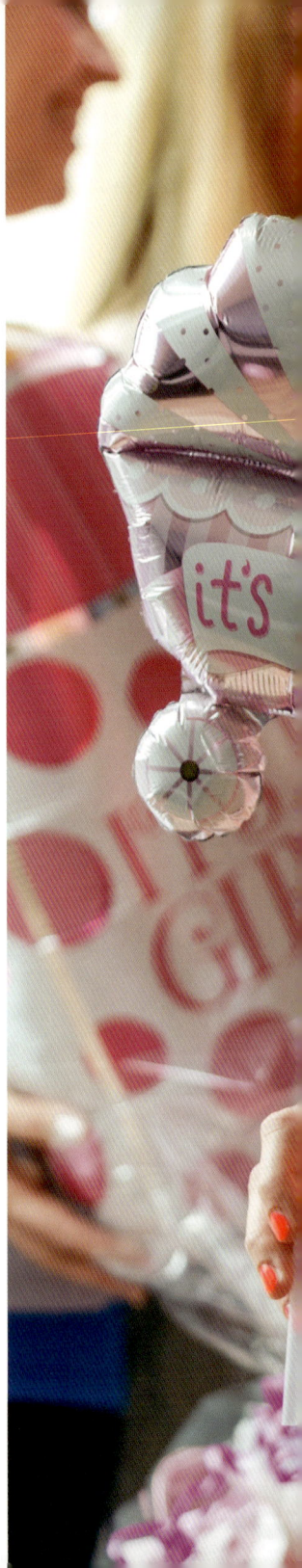

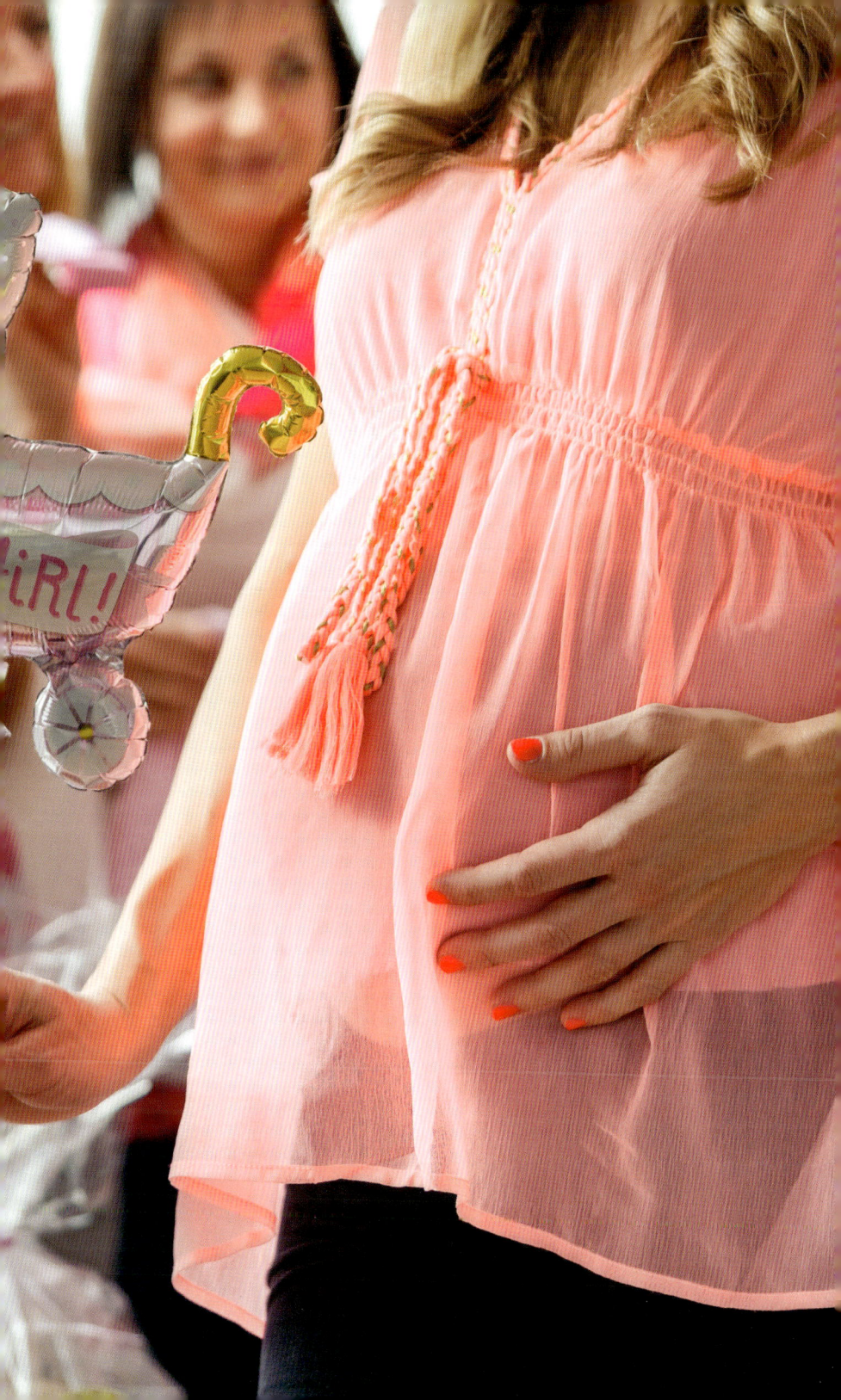

BONDING

After the birth, mom and baby need to take every opportunity to connect and bond. These oils may help encourage a stronger, deeper emotional bond.

Recommendations:
Gentle Baby · Joy
Forgiveness
TraumaLife

Topical:
- Massage 4-6 drops diluted 50:50 on neck, shoulders, and breasts (but not nipples) before feeding, up to 3 times daily.

BREAST HEALTH

Maintaining breast health is key for women who plan to breastfeed. Several studies show positive impacts on a newborn's health that may carry throughout their lives as a result of breastfeeding.

Recommendations:
Lavender · Myrrh · Melissa
Patchouli · Rosemary
Tea Tree (Melaleuca Alternifolia)
Thyme

Topical:
Dilute any of the above oils 20:80 and massage over breast (avoiding the nipples) and on Vita Flex points of the feet. The same is true for the following blends:

Breast Blend No. 1
- 3 drops Thyme
- 7 drops PanAway
- 1 teaspoon V-6 Vegetable Oil Complex

Breast Blend No. 2
- 3 drops Lemon
- 4 drops Thyme
- 2 drops Melissa
- 1 teaspoon V-6 Vegetable Oil Complex

BREECH

If a baby hasn't turned so that it is head down at the time of delivery, it can create complications. A breech birth can lead to a medical emergency for both mother and child. Skilled practitioners have been known to turn a baby successfully. If, however, such a turn isn't possible, it may be necessary for a doctor to perform a Cesarean (C-) section.

Recommendations:
Peppermint
Myrrh

Topical:

- Massage Peppermint on the top of the belly, in a half-moon, curved motion. This may help nudge the baby to turn its head down.
- Combine 5 drops Myrrh in one teaspoon carrier oil and rub on your belly in a circular motion.

BURSITIS (HIP)

Pregnancy can put a lot of strain on the areas there muscles and tendons connect with bone. The bursa are the small fluid-filled sacs that cushion those areas, and those around the hip are particularly prone to inflammation during this time.

Recommendations:
Copaiba
Deep Relief Roll-On
Dorado Azul
Frankincense · Lavender
Marjoram · PanAway
Palo Santo · Peppermint
Relieve It
Sacred Frankincense
Wintergreen

Inhalation:

- Diffuse your choice of oils for ½ hour every 4-6 hours or as desired.
- Put 2-3 drops of your chosen oil in your hands and rub them together, cup your hands over your nose, and inhale throughout the day as needed.
- Put 8-10 drops of oil on a cotton ball or tissue and put it in an air vent in your house, vehicle, hotel room, etc.
- If diffusing while sleeping, set your timer for the desired length of time for automatic shut off.

Topical:
- Apply 2-4 drops neat or diluted 50:50 on affected area or joint 3-5 times daily or as needed to soothe pain
- Apply a cold compress around affected joint 1-3 times daily.

CANKER SORES

These can flare up for a variety of reasons during pregnancy, and mostly occur for the same reasons they occur for everyone else. Canker sores often follow triggers of stress, illness, weakened immune system, certain acidic foods, scratchy foods, and visits to the dentist.

Recommendations:
Cypress · Lavender
Melrose · Melissa
Sandalwood
Thieves · Thyme

Topical:
- Gently apply 1 drop neat with fingertip to canker sore 4-8 times daily.

Ingestion & Oral:
- Gargle with Thieves mouthwash 2-4 times daily.

CAESAREAN (C-SECTION)

The World Health Organization (WHO) recommends performing this surgical procedure only when it is medically necessary, and only after other solutions have failed. In the case of breech babies WHO only recommends doing so after attempts to turn the baby are unsuccessful. It is important to prevent infection, reduce scarring, and stimulate the healing process.

Recommendations:
Geranium
Helichrysum
Lavender · Myrrh
Rose
Rose Ointment

Topical:
- Apply Helichrysum and/or Geranium on the location near the incision to reduce tissue damage and bleeding.
- Apply Lavender, Rose Ointment, Myrrh, and/or Rose to the closed incision area to assist healing.

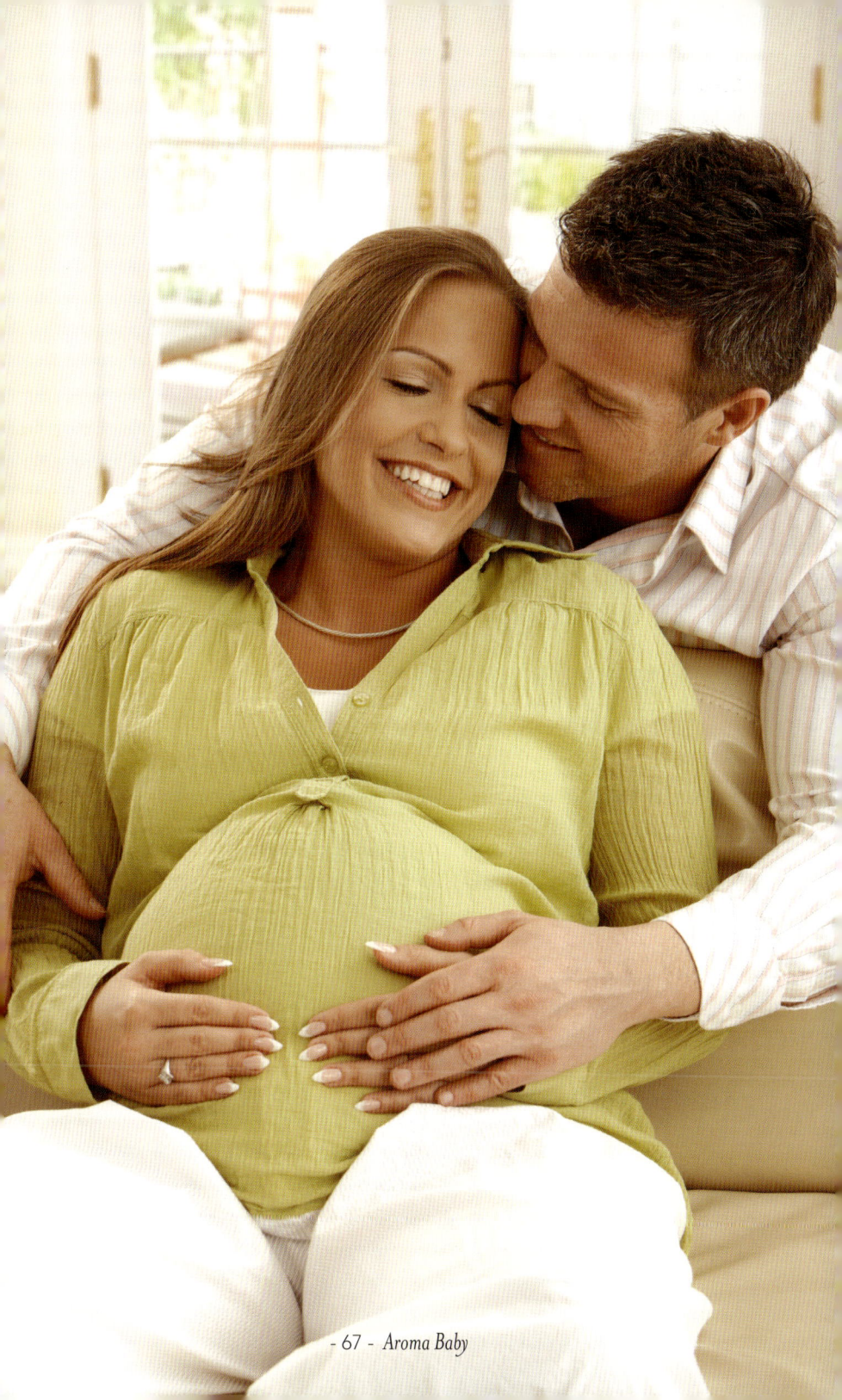

CHRONIC PAIN

If you suffer from chronic pain, chances are those symptoms will be magnified during pregnancy. This can be due to a number of factors including greater susceptibility to inflammation. Anti-inflammatory drugs and NSAIDs are generally forbidden during pregnancy so essential oils may provide a safe, healthy and effective alternative.

Recommendations:
Clove · Copaiba · Dorado Azul
Helichrysum · Idaho Blue Spruce
Idaho Balsam Fir
Oregano · Palo Santo
Peppermint
Sacred Frankincense
Frankincense · Wintergreen

Topical:
- Apply 2-4 drops diluted 50:50 on location, as needed.
- Place 1-2 drops oil with a warm compress on location, as needed.
- Sacred Frankincense or Frankincense: Take 1 capsule daily.

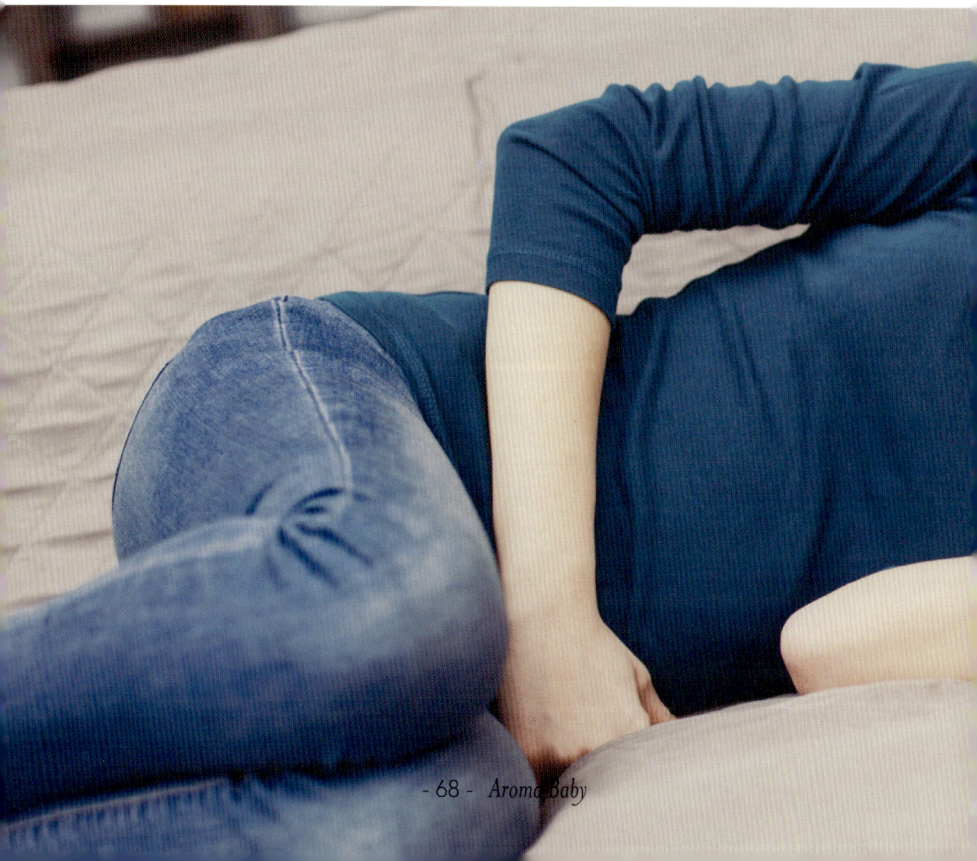

COLD SORES

Many pregnant mothers experience an outbreak of cold sores during their pregnancy. Many women feel it's important to use natural alternatives to treat their cold sores and avoid taking prescription medications.

Topical:
- Apply single oils or blends neat or diluted, depending on the oils being used.
- Apply 1 drop neat as soon as the cold sore appears. Repeat 5-10 times daily.
- If needed, dilute 50:50 with V-6 Vegetable Oil Complex or Rose Ointment to reduce discomfort of drying skin after applying essential oils to an open sore.

Recommendations:
Lavender · Melissa · Melrose
Mountain Savory
Oregano · Peppermint
Ravintsara · Sandalwood
Tea Tree (Melaleuca Alternifolia)
Thieves · Thyme

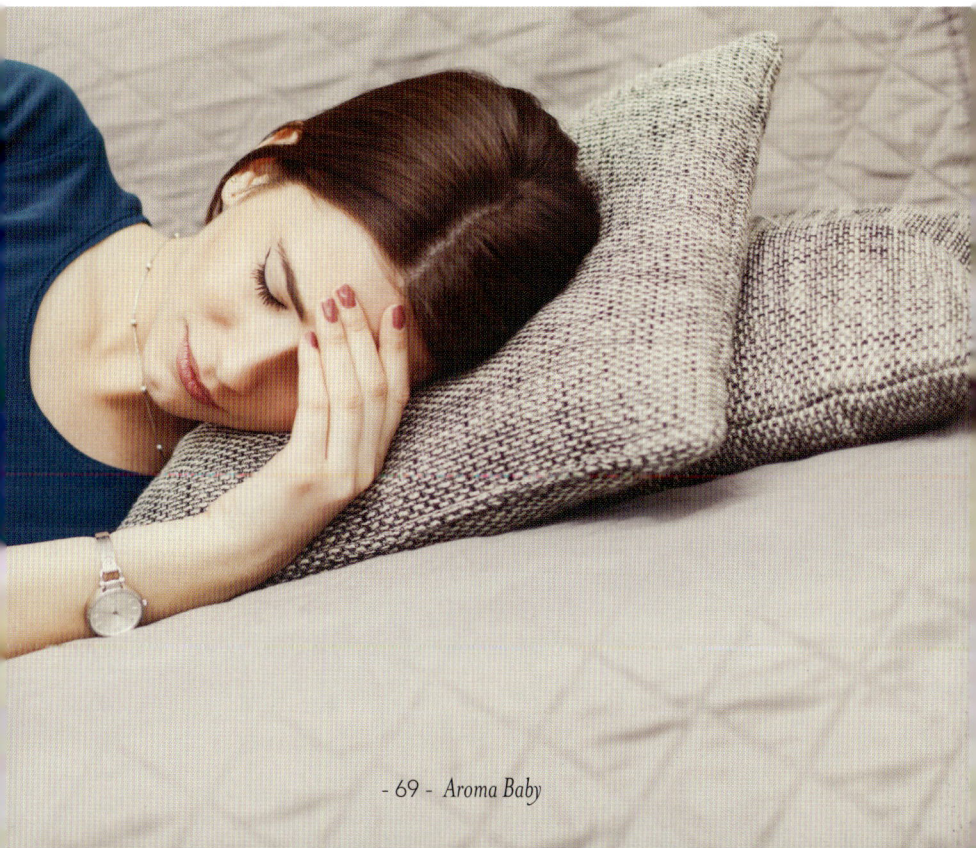

CONCENTRATION

Many women report that it's harder to concentrate or think clearly while they are pregnant. This may be a result of different hormones or simply because they have more decisions and concerns to cope with during pregnancy. Thankfully, essential oils have time-proven effects on memory and concentration.

Recommendations:
Brain Power · Clarity · Basil
Bergamot · Dorado Azul
Frankincense · Lemon
Peppermint · Rosemary
Sacred Frankincense

Inhalation:

- Diffuse your choice of oils for ½ hour every 4-6 hours or as desired.
- Put 2-3 drops of your chosen oil in your hands and rub them together, cup your hands over your nose, and inhale throughout the day as needed.
- Put 8-10 drops of oil on a cotton ball or tissue and put it in an air vent in your house, vehicle, hotel room, etc.
- If diffusing while sleeping, set your timer for the desired length of time for automatic shut off.

Topical:

- Apply 1-2 drops neat directly onto the brain reflex centers 2-4 times daily, as needed. These points include the forehead, temples, and mastoids (the bones just behind the ears). Apply oils and mild, direct pressure to the brainstem area (center top of neck at base of skull) and work down the spine.
- Apply 1-2 drops neat to Vita Flex brain points on feet 1-2 times daily.

CONGESTION

This may be result of allergies, flu, or the common cold. In any case, many essential oils can prevent the need for harsh chemical compounds in over-the-counter drugs and may be just as effective in treating the symptoms.

Recommendations:
Blue Cypress · Dorado Azul
Eucalyptus Blue · Peppermint
Peppermint Vitality
Rosemary · Rosemary Vitality
Thyme · Thyme Vitality
Thieves · Thieves Vitality
Ravintsara

Inhalation:
- Diffuse your choice of oils for ½ hour every 4-6 hours or as desired.
- Put 2-3 drops of your chosen oil in your hands and rub them together, cup your hands over your nose, and inhale throughout the day as needed.
- Put 8-10 drops of oil on a cotton ball or tissue and put it in an air vent in your house, vehicle, hotel room, etc.
- If diffusing while sleeping, set your timer for the desired length of time for automatic shut off.

Topical:
- Apply 1-2 drops diluted 50:50 just under jawbone on right and left sides 4-8 times daily.
- You may also apply 2-3 drops on the Vita Flex points of the feet.

Oral:
- Gargle 2-5 times daily with water that contains 1-2 drops of any of the above essential oils. Spit it out. Rinse.
- Apply 1-2 drops diluted 50:50 of Thieves Vitality at the very back of the tongue and hold it in the mouth, mixing it with saliva for several minutes, and then swallow. This can be very effective if started at the very first indication of infection and repeated 3-4 times for the first hour, then once an hour until symptoms subside.
- Spray inside mouth with Thieves Spray as often as desired.

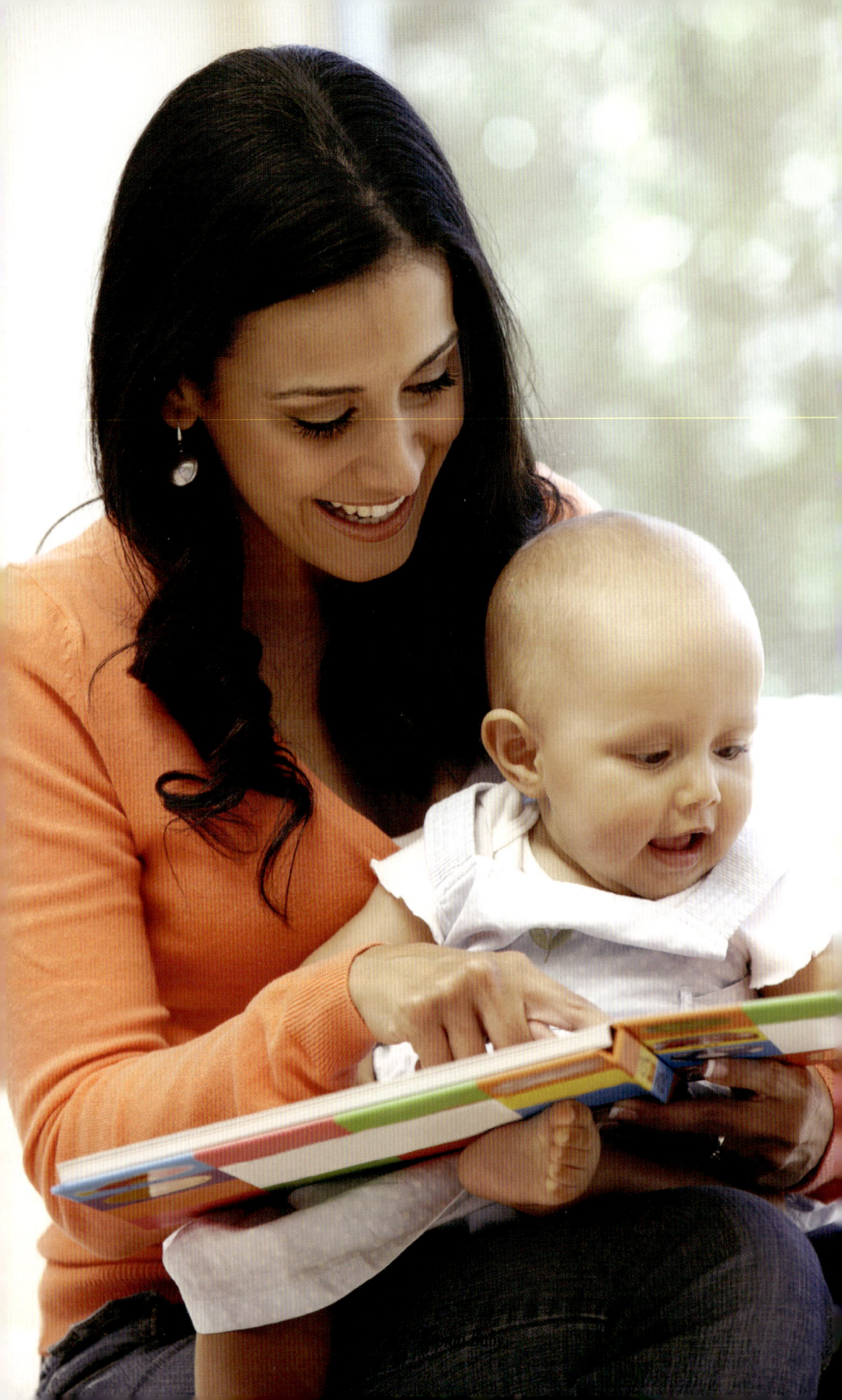

CONSTIPATION

While this may not ordinarily be a problem for most women under regular circumstances, it is common for women to develop a case of constipation at some time during their pregnancy. This can be due to a change in fluid intake, the need for more hydration during pregnancy, and the pressure the uterus places on the abdomen. A good supplement regimen may be just the thing to keep you in the clear:

Recommendations:
Ginger · Ginger Vitality
Fennel · Fennel Vitality
Tarragon · Tarragon
Vitality Peppermint
Peppermint Vitality

- Essentialzymes[4]: Take 3-6 tablets 3 times daily.
- ComforTone: Start with 1 capsule and increase the next day to 2 capsules. Continue to increase 1 capsule each day until bowels start moving.
- ICP: 1 week after ComforTone, start with 1 tablespoon ICP 2 times daily and then increase to 3 times daily up to 2 tablespoons 3 times daily.
- Balance Complete: 3 scoops daily or as needed.
- Drink at least ½ cup unsweetened cherry juice, prune juice, pineapple juice, or other raw fruit and vegetable juices each morning.
- Drink 8 glasses of pure water daily.

Inhalation:
- Diffuse your choice of oils for ½ hour every 4-6 hours or as desired.
- Put 2-3 drops of your chosen oil in your hands and rub them together, cup your hands over your nose, and inhale throughout the day as needed.
- Put 8-10 drops of oil on a cotton ball or tissue and put it in an air vent in your house, vehicle, hotel room, etc.
- If diffusing while sleeping, set your timer for the desired length of time for automatic shut off.

Topical:
- Apply 6-10 drops neat or diluted 50:50 on stomach area as desired.
- Applying a single drop under the nose is helpful and refreshing.
- Place a warm compress with 1-3 drops of recommended oil over the stomach area and Vita Flex points of the feet.

Ingestion & Oral:

- Take 1 capsule with desired Vitality line oil 2 times daily.
- Put 2-3 drops of Vitality line oil in a spoonful of Blue Agave, Yacon Syrup, maple syrup, coconut oil, milk, etc.
- Put the desired amount of oils in a glass of rice milk, almond milk, goat milk, carrot juice, NingXia Red, or even water and then drink it.

CONJUNCTIVITIS (PINK EYE)

Being in settings with children can put you at higher risk, since this condition is so contagious and spreads so easily with contact. Washing your hands thoroughly is the best prevention, but essential oils can help with some of the symptoms until the infection runs its course.

> *Recommendations:*
> *Myrrh*
> *Lavender*
> *Vetiver*

Inhalation:

- Diffuse your choice of oils for ½ hour every 4-6 hours or as desired.
- Put 2-3 drops of your chosen oil in your hands and rub them together, cup your hands over your nose, and inhale throughout the day as needed.
- Put 8-10 drops of oil on a cotton ball or tissue and put it in an air vent in your house, vehicle, hotel room, etc.
- If diffusing while sleeping, set your timer for the desired length of time for automatic shut off.

Topical:

- Apply 2-4 drops diluted 20:80 in a wide circle around the eye 1-3 times daily, being careful not to get any oil in the eyes or on the eyelids. This may also help with puffiness.
- Apply on temples and eye Vita Flex points on the feet and hands (the undersides of your two largest toes and your index and middle fingers).

Note: If essential oils should ever accidentally get into the eyes, dilute with V-6 Vegetable Oil Complex or other pure vegetable oil. Never rinse with water. However, the essential oils will not cause any damage and will slowly stop burning.

COUGH

A cough may be simply caused by a tickle in the throat or it may be the sign of something more serious. If it persists and is accompanied by fever, it's important to seek medical attention. These suggestions are for managing a minor cough with a determinable cause.

Recommendations:
Idaho Ponderosa Pine
Basil · Lavender · Nutmeg
Peppermint · Oregano
Rosemary
Tea Tree
(Melaleuca Alternifolia)
Thyme · Wintergreen

Inhalation:
- Diffuse your choice of oils for 15 minutes, alternating between singles and blends 3-10 times daily as needed.
- Put 2-3 drops of your chosen oil in your hands and rub them together, cup your hands over your nose, and inhale throughout the day as needed.
- Put 8-10 drops of oil on a cotton ball or tissue and put it in an air vent in your house, vehicle, hotel room, etc.
- If diffusing while sleeping, set your timer for the desired length of time for automatic shut off.
- Add a few drops of oil to a bowl of boiling water. Position the face above the bowl and drape a towel over the head to create a vaporizing effect. Repeat 2-4 times daily.

Topical:
- Apply 2-4 drops diluted 50:50 on neck and chest as needed.
- Massage 2-4 drops of oil neat on the soles of the feet and on Vita Flex points just before bedtime. Children may especially benefit from this application.
- Place a warm compress with 1-2 drops of chosen oil on the neck, chest, and upper back area 1-3 times daily.

Ingestion & Oral:
Mix 10 drops Myrrh and 1 drop Peppermint in water and gargle.

CRAMPS (ABDOMINAL)

Some abdominal cramps are common and usually they are benign. In some rarer cases, however, abdominal aches and pains can imply something more serious. Cramps can be simply from constipation, the uterus expanding, the round ligaments expanding, or Braxton Hicks. It's important to pay attention to cramps. If they are more severe, they may be a sign of an ectopic pregnancy, preterm labor, placental abruption, a urinary tract infection (UTI), preeclampsia, or miscarriage. Any of these would be reason to seek immediate medical attention.

Recommendations:
Ginger · Ginger Vitality
Fennel · Fennel Vitality
Tarragon
Tarragon Vitality
Peppermint
Peppermint Vitality

Inhalation:
- Diffuse your choice of oils for ½ hour every 4-6 hours or as desired.
- Put 2-3 drops of your chosen oil in your hands and rub them together, cup your hands over your nose, and inhale throughout the day as needed.
- Put 8-10 drops of oil on a cotton ball or tissue and put it in an air vent in your house, vehicle, hotel room, etc.
- If diffusing while sleeping, set your timer for the desired length of time for automatic shut off.

Topical:
- Apply 6-10 drops neat or diluted 50:50 on stomach area as desired.
- Applying a single drop under the nose is helpful and refreshing.
- Place a warm compress with 1-3 drops of recommended oil over the stomach area and Vita Flex points of the feet.

Ingestion & Oral:
- Take 1 capsule with desired Vitality line oil 2 times daily.
- Put 2-3 drops of Vitality line oil in a spoonful of Blue Agave, Yacon Syrup, maple syrup, coconut oil, milk, etc.
- Put the desired amount of oils in a glass of rice milk, almond milk, goat milk, carrot juice, NingXia Red, or even water and then drink it.

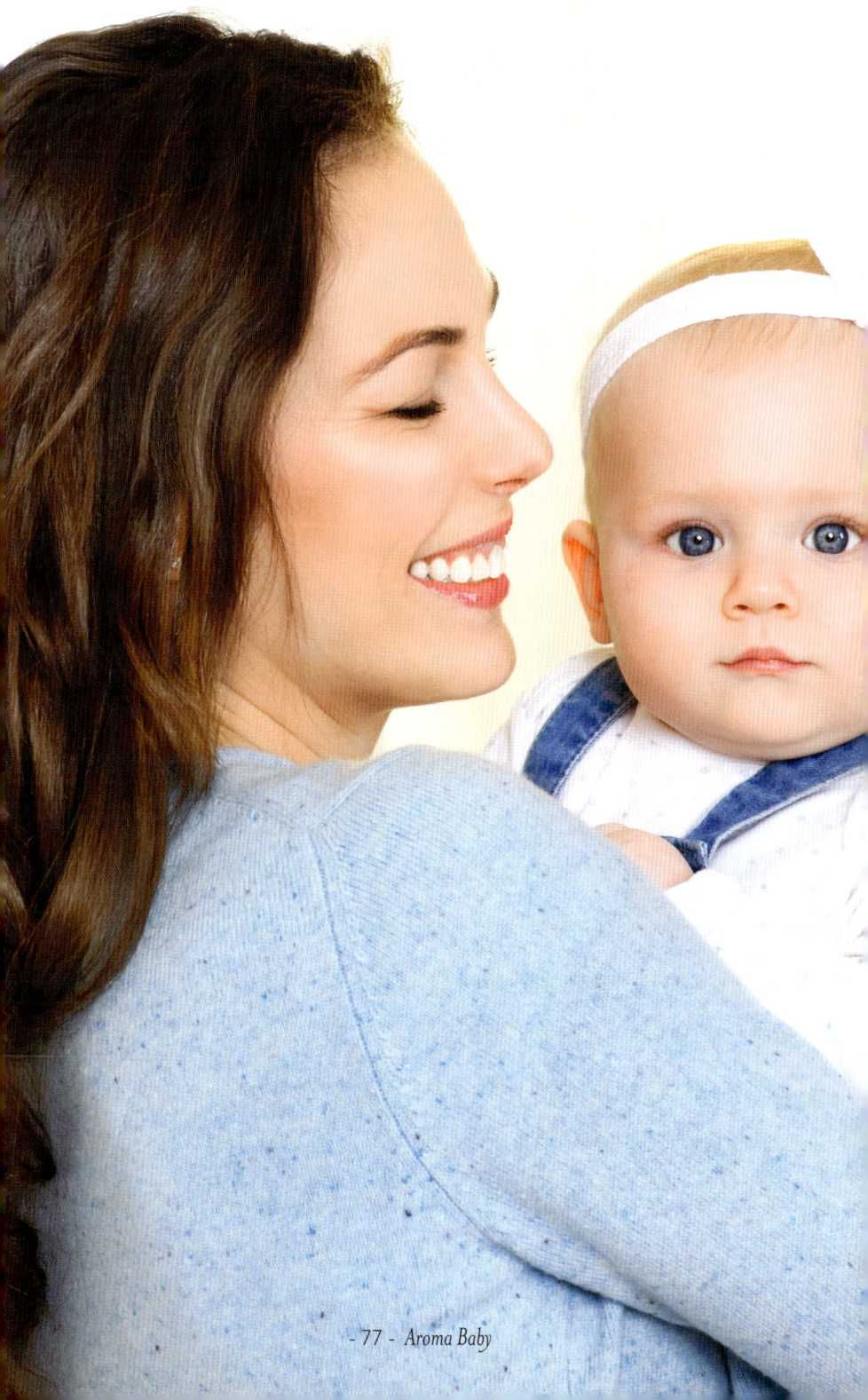

DELIVERY

Once labor has begun, this Labor Blend can help support a healthy delivery. It's important only to use this blend during delivery, not any time beforehand:

Labor Blend
(Use only after labor has started.)

- 5 drops Ylang Ylang
  (or Amazonian Ylang Ylang)
- 4 drops Helichrysum
- 2 drops Fennel
- 2 drops Peppermint
- 2 drops Clary Sage

Recommendations:
Gentle Baby · Geranium
German Chamomile
Forgiveness · Grounding
Highest Potential · Lavender Myrrh
· Rose · Joy · Helichrysum
Neroli · Peace & Calming
Sacred Mountain · Sandalwood
Valor · Valor Roll-On
White Angelica · Ylang Ylang

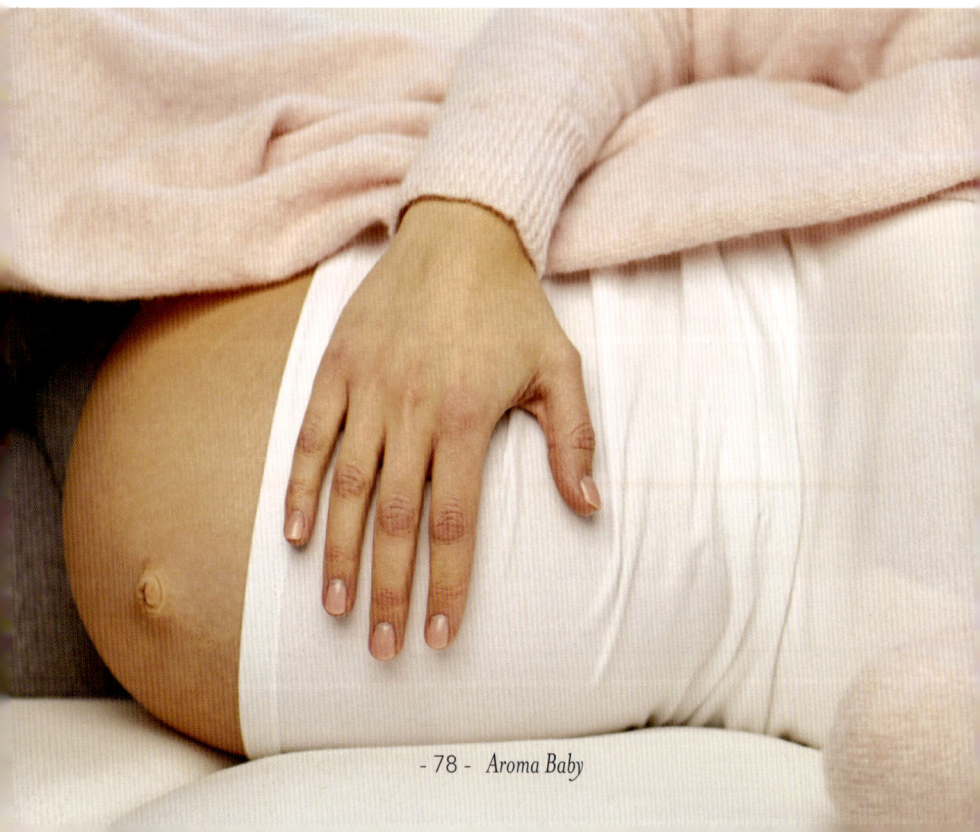

Inhalation:
- Diffuse your choice of oils for ½ hour every 4-6 hours or as desired.
- Put 2-3 drops of your chosen oil in your hands and rub them together, cup your hands over your nose, and inhale throughout the day as needed.
- Put 8-10 drops of oil on a cotton ball or tissue and put it in an air vent in your house, vehicle, hotel room, etc.
- If diffusing while sleeping, set your timer for the desired length of time for automatic shut off.
- Diffuse Gentle Baby, Joy, or Valor to reduce stress before and after the birth. Expectant fathers will also find this helps to reduce anxiety during delivery.

Topical:
- Massage 2-4 drops Labor Blend from above diluted 50:50 on reproductive Vita Flex points on the sides of the ankles. Apply ONLY after labor has started.
- Massage 2-4 drops Labor Blend from above on lower stomach and lower back.

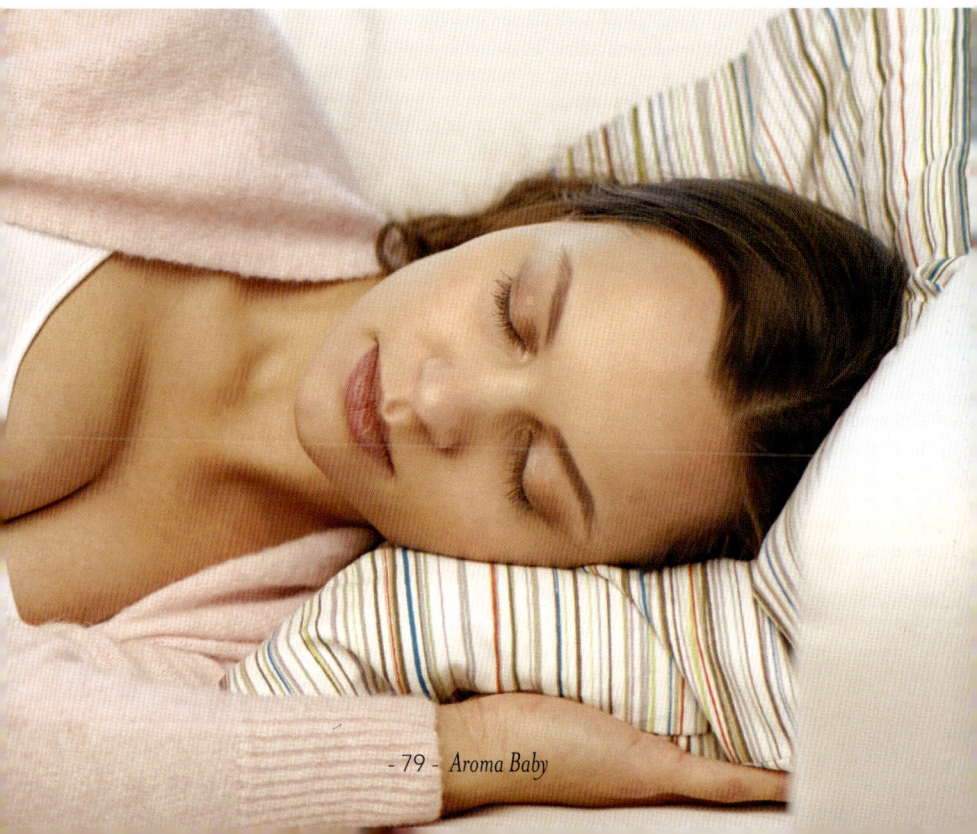

DE QUERVAIN'S TENOSYNOVITIS
(THUMB & WRIST PAIN)

This is also known as mother's wrist or mommy's thumb. Symptoms usually improve naturally over 4-6 weeks. The only course of action is to treat the symptoms. Thankfully, this blend can help:

Recommendations:
Aroma Siez · Copaiba
Deep Relief Roll-On
Dorado Azul · Idaho Blue Spruce
Helichrysum · Idaho Balsam Fir
Lemongrass · Marjoram
Palo Santo · PanAway
Peppermint · Relieve It
Wintergreen

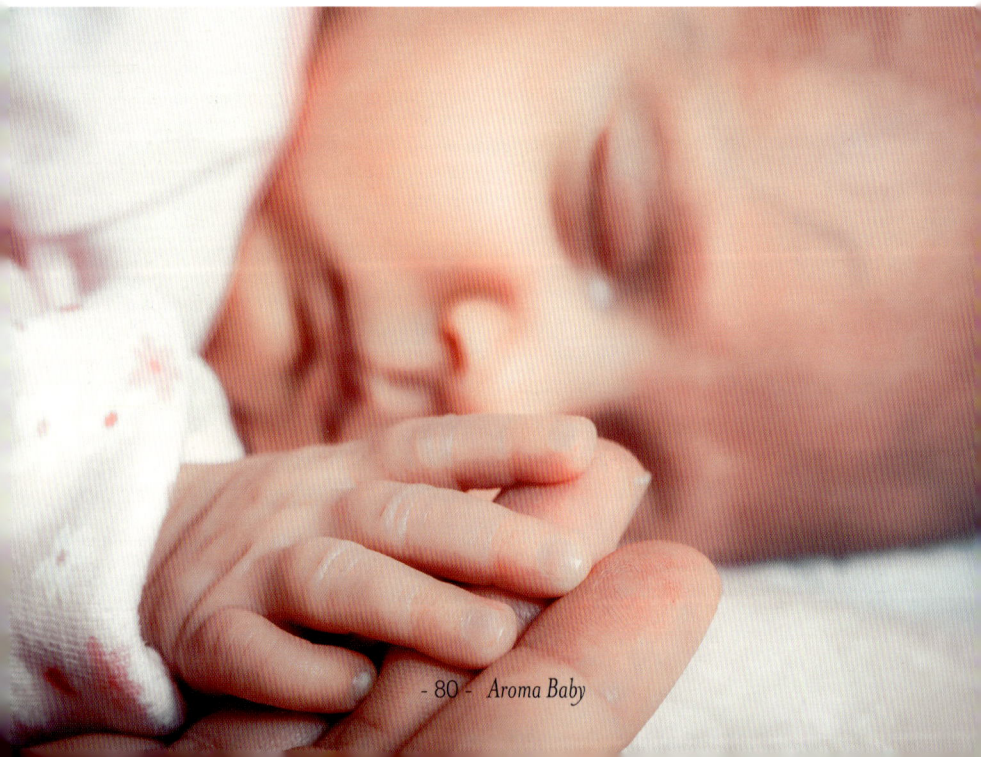

Wrist/Thumb Relief Blend
- 12 drops Wintergreen
- 10 drops Marjoram
- 9 drops Lemongrass

Topical:
- Apply neat or diluted 50:50 on location 3-6 times daily.
- Massage 4-6 drops of oil on affected area. For swelling, elevate and apply ice packs.
- Place a cold compress with 1-2 drops of chosen oil in Ortho Ease or Ortho Sport Massage Oil on area 2-4 times daily.

DIABETES (GESTATIONAL)

It's important to manage gestational diabetes to protect both you and your baby. The only way to be sure you have it (or to rule it out) is by screening during pregnancy. Be sure to consult a medical professional as you look for ways to manage your blood sugar.

> **Recommendations:**
> Cinnamon Bark Vitality
> Coriander
> DiGize Vitality
> Ocotea

Ingestion:
- Take 2 capsules 50:50 Ocotea and Coriander 2 times daily.
- Take 2 capsules 50:50 Cinnamon Bark Vitality and DiGize Vitality 2 times daily.
- Put 2-3 drops of Vitality line oil in a spoonful of Blue Agave, Yacon Syrup, maple syrup, coconut oil, milk, etc.
- Put the desired amount of oils in a glass of rice milk, almond milk, goat milk, carrot juice, NingXia Red, or even water and then drink it.

DIARRHEA

When you take measures to prevent constipation, you may just go the other way. Diarrhea can also cause cramping and discomfort. The important thing is to stay hydrated with a balance of electrolytes to keep you and the baby in tip-top shape.

> **Recommendations:**
> DiGize · DiGize Vitality
> Ginger · Ginger Vitality
> Lavender · Lavender
> Vitality Peppermint
> Peppermint Vitality
> Rosemary
> Rosemary Vitality

Topical:
- Dilute 50:50 and apply 6-10 drops over stomach area 2 times daily.
- Apply a warm compress 1-2 times daily.
- Apply 1-3 drops on stomach Vita Flex points of feet.

Ingestion & Oral:
- Take 1 capsule with desired Vitality line oil 2 times daily.
- Put 2-3 drops of Vitality line oil in a spoonful of Blue Agave, Yacon Syrup, maple syrup, coconut oil, milk, etc.

- Put the desired amount of oils in a glass of rice milk, almond milk, goat milk, carrot juice, NingXia Red, or even water and then drink it.

DILATION (DELAYED)

This suggestion is only for when labor has begun and the professional health practitioner suggests that dilation needs to progress.

Recommendations:
Clary Sage
Fennel
Helichrysum
Peppermint
Ylang Ylang

Labor Blend
(Use only after labor has started.)
- 5 drops Ylang Ylang
  (or Amazonian Ylang Ylang)
- 4 drops Helichrysum
- 2 drops Fennel
- 2 drops Peppermint
- 2 drops Clary Sage

Topical:
- Massage 2-4 drops Labor Blend from above diluted 50:50 on reproductive Vita Flex points on the sides of the ankles. Apply ONLY after labor has started.
- Massage 2-4 drops Labor Blend from above on lower stomach and lower back.

Ingestion & Oral:
- Take 1 capsule with 2-4 drops of Clary Sage. Or, put 2-3 drops of Vitality line oil in a spoonful of Blue Agave, Yacon Syrup, maple syrup, coconut oil, milk, etc. Observe dilation and progress. Repeat after 2 hours if necessary.

DISINFECTION

Throughout your pregnancy, Thieves products will be helpful in cleaning/sanitizing surfaces as well as foods. Thieves Spray and Thieves Household Cleaner are good for general household cleaning. Thieves Fruit & Veggie Soak is great for cleaning foods. Thieves essential oil is great for the body and diffusing, and Thieves Vitality works wonders in supporting your healthy immune system.

Recommendations:
Thieves
Thieves Fruit & Veggie Soak
Thieves Household Cleaner
Thieves Spray
Thieves Vitality
Thieves Wipes

Inhalation:
- Diffuse Thieves for 1 hour 3 times daily.
- Put 2-3 drops of Thieves oil in your hands and rub them together, cup your hands over your nose, and inhale throughout the day as needed.
- Put 8-10 drops of Thieves on a cotton ball or tissue and put it in an air vent in your house, vehicle, hotel room, etc.
- If diffusing while sleeping, set your timer for the desired length of time for automatic shut off.

Topical:
- Apply 3-5 drops diluted 50:50 on the bottoms of the feet and on carotid artery spots under the earlobes.
- Use Thieves Wipes, Thieves Household Cleaner, Thieves Spray, and Thieves Fruit & Veggie Soak as directed on the label.

Ingestion & Oral:
- Take 1 capsule with Thieves Vitality 2 times daily.
- Put 2-3 drops of Thieves Vitality in a spoonful of Blue Agave, Yacon Syrup, maple syrup, coconut oil, milk, etc.
- Put the desired amount of Thieves Vitality in a glass of rice milk, almond milk, goat milk, carrot juice, NingXia Red, or even water and then drink it.

DIZZINESS

Dizziness by itself is really a symptom of something else. It is a common result of low blood sugar, dehydration, low blood pressure, getting up too quickly—all of which happen all the time during pregnancy.

Recommendations:
Basil · Brain Power
Cardamom · Citrus Fresh
Clarity · Frankincense
Grounding · Ocotea
Sandalwood · Tangerine

Inhalation:

- Diffuse your choice of oils for ½ hour every 4-6 hours or as desired.
- Put 2-3 drops of your chosen oil in your hands and rub them together, cup your hands over your nose, and inhale throughout the day as needed.
- Put 8-10 drops of oil on a cotton ball or tissue and put it in an air vent in your house, vehicle, hotel room, etc.
- If diffusing while sleeping, set your timer for the desired length of time for automatic shut off.

Topical:

- Apply 1-2 drops neat (undiluted) on temples and back of neck, as desired.
- Applying a single drop under the nose is helpful and refreshing.
- Massage 2-4 drops of oil neat on the soles of the feet just before bedtime.

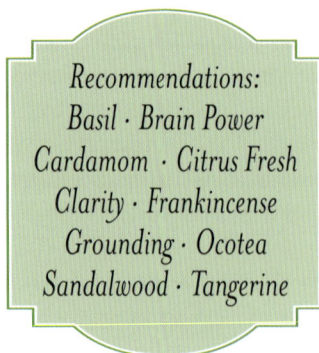

ECZEMA / DERMATITIS

About 80 of women who report pregnancy eczema never experienced it until they became pregnant. This may be due to the stress that comes with pregnancy, which happens to be the primary trigger. Rather than taking cortisone or other corticosteroids, essential oils offer a safer, more natural alternative.

Recommendations:
Geranium
Lavender · Melrose
Myrrh · Purification
Rose

Topical:

- Apply 1-2 drops diluted 50:50 on location as needed.

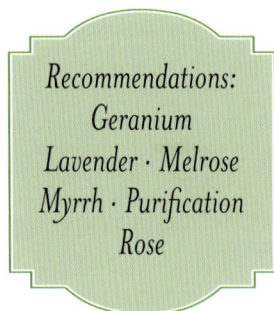

EDEMA (WATER RETENTION)

Most women experience some degree of water retention in the form of swollen feet, hands, fingers, legs, ankles, neck, and even face. Much of this is normal because the fluids in your body increase to nurture both your tissues and those of the baby.

Edema Blend (General)
- 10 drops Wintergreen
- 8 drops Tangerine
- 6 drops Fennel
- 4 drops Juniper
- 3 drops Patchouli

Edema Blend (Morning)
- 10 drops Tangerine
- 10 drops Cypress

Recommendations:
Aroma Life · Cypress
DiGize · Fennel · Geranium
Grapefruit · Helichrysum
Lavender · Patchouli
Peppermint · Tangerine
Wintergreen

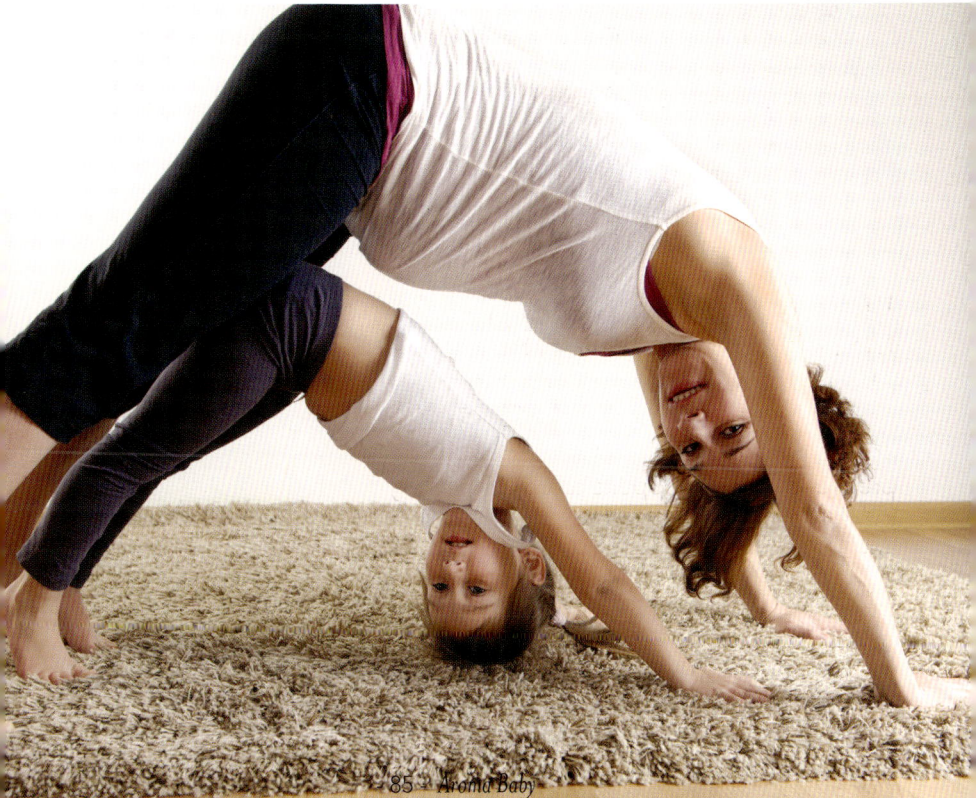

Edema Blend (Evening)
- 8 drops Geranium
- 5 drops Cypress
- 5 drops Helichrysum or Grapefruit

Topical:
- Apply 1-3 drops diluted 50:50 on affected area 2-3 times daily.
- Place a cold compress with 1-2 drops of chosen oil 1-2 times daily on the area.
- Massage 1-3 drops on bladder Vita Flex point on foot.
- Massage 15-20 drops of the General Edema Blend diluted 60:40 in V-6 Vegetable Oil Complex or other massage oil on legs, working from the feet up to the thighs. Do this for 1 week.
- Massage 15-20 drops of Morning Edema Blend diluted 60:40 in V-6 Vegetable Oil Complex or other massage oil on legs, working from the feet up to the thighs. Do this in the morning for 1 week. Repeat the same process in the evening with the Evening Edema Blend.

Ingestion & Oral:
- Take 1 capsule with desired Vitality line oil 2 times daily.
- Put 2-3 drops of Vitality line oil in a spoonful of Blue Agave, Yacon Syrup, maple syrup, coconut oil, milk, etc.
- Put the desired amount of oils in a glass of rice milk, almond milk, goat milk, carrot juice, NingXia Red, or even water and then drink it.

EMOTIONAL BALANCE

Pregnancy can be an emotional roller-coaster ride. Not only are your hormones changing your comfort and how you feel, but several events during pregnancy may cause you stress, anxiety, or even fear. It is important to keep your emotions in balance as best you can for the most ideal outcome for your and your baby.

Recommendations:
Forgiveness · Joy
Peace & Calming
Present Time
Stress Away Roll-On
Surrender

Inhalation:
- Diffuse your choice of oils for ½ hour every 4-6 hours or as desired.

- Put 2-3 drops of your chosen oil in your hands and rub them together, cup your hands over your nose, and inhale throughout the day as needed.
- Put 8-10 drops of oil on a cotton ball or tissue and put it in an air vent in your house, vehicle, hotel room, etc.
- If diffusing while sleeping, set your timer for the desired length of time for automatic shut off.

Topical:
- Apply 1-2 drops neat (undiluted) on temples and back of neck, as desired.
- Applying a single drop under the nose is helpful and refreshing.
- Massage 2-4 drops of oil neat on the soles of the feet just before bedtime.

EPISIOTOMY

Preparing your perineal tissue in advance of labor may allow the tissue to flex and expand during birth. Using several essential oils can condition the area so that an episiotomy is unnecessary. Or if having one becomes necessary, the procedure may be much less invasive, and the healing/recovery may be enhanced.

Recommendations:
ClaraDerm · Gentle Baby
Geranium · Helichrysum
Lavender · Myrrh
Peace & Calming
Rose · Rose Ointment

Topical:
- Apply 1-2 drops neat or undiluted as desired.
- Apply 1-3 drops diluted 50:50 on affected area 2-3 times daily.

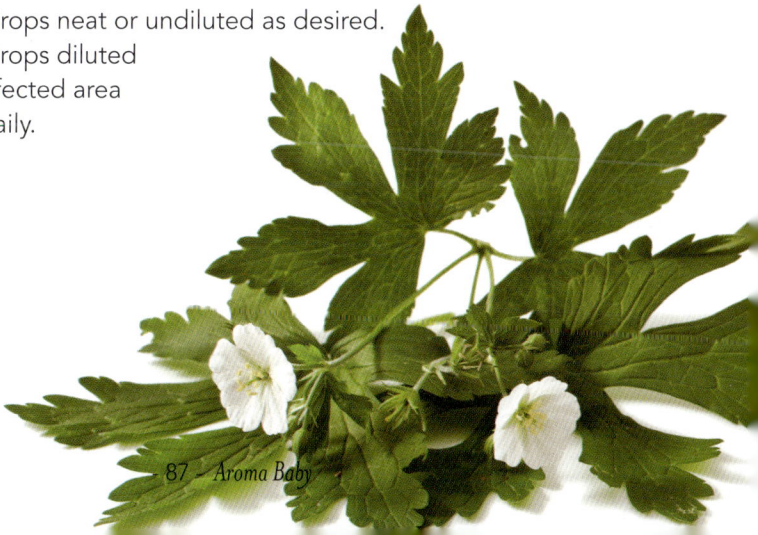

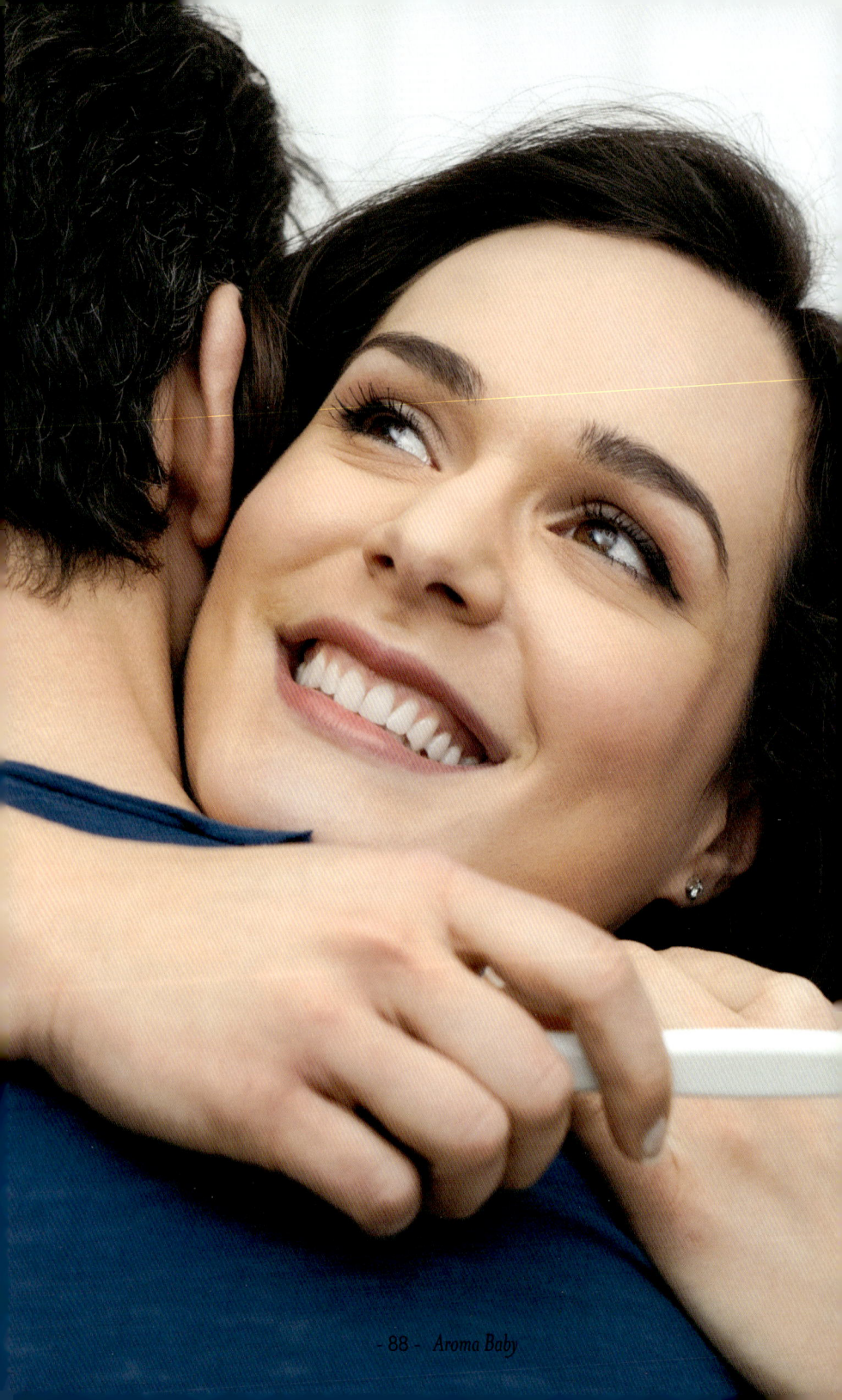

EYE HEALTH

Taking care of your eyes is important. It's also very important when it comes to your infant and toddler. Children, especially babies, rub their eyes without any regard for how clean their fingers and hands are. These recommendations are for moms, but we've included infant-specific and toddler-specific instructions in the following sections.

Recommendations:
Cypress · Frankincense
Idaho Blue Spruce
Lavender
Sacred Frankincense
Sacred Mountain

Eye Blend
- 10 drops Lemongrass
- 5 drops Cypress
- 3 drops Eucalyptus Radiata
- 2 drops Sacred Frankincense or Frankincense

Topical:
- Mix the Eye Blend with a little V-6 Vegetable Oil Complex and apply around the eyes, being careful not to touch the eyes. It is best at night because the eyes may water.
- Massage 3-6 drops using the Vita Flex technique on the bottoms of feet 2 times daily.
- Rubbing 1 drop of Lavender oil over the bridge of the nose 2 times daily has been reported to help in some cases.

FEVER

During pregnancy, many women seek alternatives to NSAIDs (non-steroidal anti-inflammatory drugs) when possible. Fever can be a symptom of serious health issues and infection. Be sure to consult a medical professional when you experience fever during pregnancy. The following options may be useful in helping to manage minor fever while reducing the use of NSAIDs.

Recommendations:
Copaiba · Dorado Azul
ImmuPower · Lavender
Lavender Vitality
Melrose · Myrrh
Nutmeg · Nutmeg Vitality
Thieves · Thieves Vitality

Inhalation:
- Diffuse your choice of oils for ½ hour every 4-6 hours or as desired.
- Put 2-3 drops of your chosen oil in your hands and rub them together, cup your hands over your nose, and inhale throughout the day as needed.
- Put 8-10 drops of oil on a cotton ball or tissue and put it in an air vent in your house, vehicle, hotel room, etc.
- If diffusing while sleeping, set your timer for the desired length of time for automatic shut off.

Topical:
- Apply 2-3 drops diluted 50:50 to forehead, temples, and back of neck.
- You may also apply 2-3 drops on the Vita Flex liver point of the right foot.

Ingestion & Oral:
- Take 1 capsule with desired Vitality line oil 2 times daily.
- Put 2-3 drops of Vitality line oil in a spoonful of Blue Agave, Yacon Syrup, maple syrup, coconut oil, milk, etc.
- Put the desired amount of oils in a glass of rice milk, almond milk, goat milk, carrot juice, NingXia Red, or even water and then drink it.

FLATULENCE (GAS)

This can be a natural result of the slower digestive system caused by higher levels of progesterone during pregnancy.

Recommendations:
Clove · Clove Vitality · DiGize
DiGize Vitality · Ginger
Ginger Vitality · Fennel
Fennel Vitality · Peppermint
Peppermint Vitality
Longevity · Nutmeg
Nutmeg Vitality · Oregano
Oregano Vitality · Thyme
Thieves · Thieves Vitality
Thyme Vitality

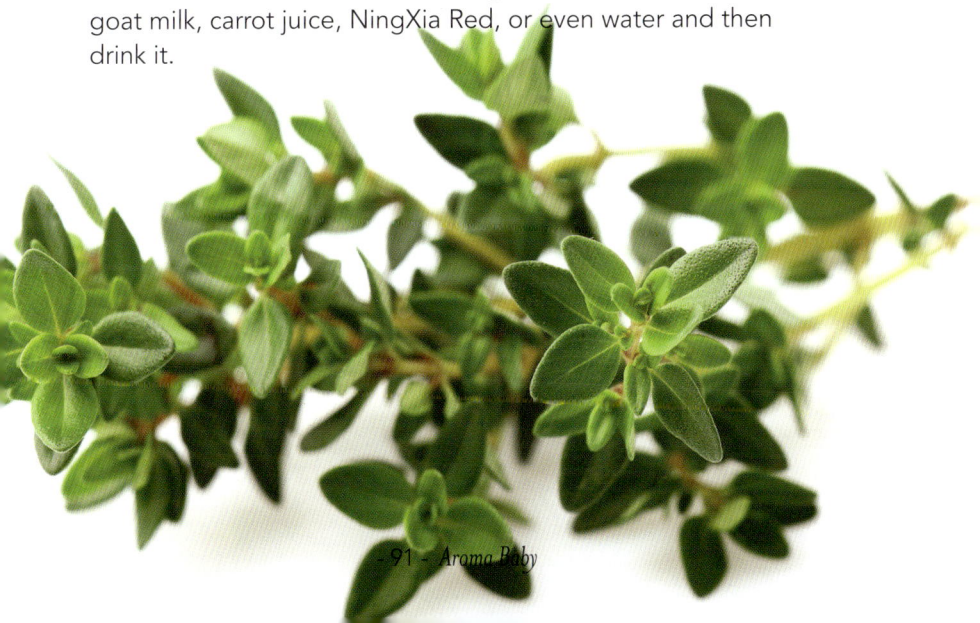

Inhalation:
- Diffuse your choice of oils for ½ hour every 4-6 hours or as desired.
- Applying a single drop under the nose is helpful and refreshing.
- Put 2-3 drops of your chosen oil in your hands and rub them together, cup your hands over your nose, and inhale throughout the day as needed.
- Put 8-10 drops of oil on a cotton ball or tissue and put it in an air vent in your house, vehicle, hotel room, etc.
- If diffusing while sleeping, set your timer for the desired length of time for automatic shut off.

Ingestion & Oral:
- Take 1 capsule with desired oil 2 times daily.
- Put 2-3 drops of oil in a spoonful of Blue Agave, Yacon Syrup, maple syrup, coconut oil, milk, etc.
- Put the desired amount of oils in a glass of rice milk, almond milk, goat milk, carrot juice, NingXia Red, or even water and then drink it.

GERD (GASTROESOPHAGEAL REFLUX DISEASE)

Gastroesophageal Reflux Disease is a serious acid condition. If allowed to go untreated for long periods of time, it may lead to certain types of throat cancer. During pregnancy, the change in hormones may relax the muscles around the lower esophageal sphincter (LES) and cause some acid to escape the stomach and return to the throat. If you suffer from GERD before pregnancy, you may consider avoiding your strong medications (both over the counter and prescription). Essential oils may be able to help alleviate symptoms until you've completed your pregnancy.

Recommendations:
Copaiba · DiGize
DiGize Vitality · Lemon
Lemon Vitality · Lemongrass
Lemongrass Vitality
Melrose · Myrtle
Myrrh · Patchouli
Peppermint · Thieves
Thieves Vitality

Inhalation:
- Diffuse your choice of oils for ½ hour every 4-6 hours or as desired.
- Put 2-3 drops of your chosen oil in your hands and rub them together, cup your hands over your nose, and inhale throughout the day as needed.
- Put 8-10 drops of oil on a cotton ball or tissue and put it in an air vent in your house, vehicle, hotel room, etc.
- If diffusing while sleeping, set your timer for the desired length of time for automatic shut off.

Topical:
Any calming oil applied through massage may help to decrease stress and bring a relaxing, balanced atmosphere.

Ingestion & Oral:
- Take 1 capsule with desired oil 3 times daily for 20 days.
- Put 2-3 drops of oil in a spoonful of Blue Agave, Yacon Syrup, maple syrup, coconut oil, milk, etc.
- Put the desired amount of oils in a glass of rice milk, almond milk, goat milk, carrot juice, NingXia Red, or even water and then drink it.

HEADACHES

Headaches are most often caused by hormone shifts, circulatory problems, stress, sugar imbalance (hypoglycemia), structural (spinal) misalignments, and blood pressure—all of which can be issues during pregnancy. If you suspect an increase in blood pressure or blood sugar, be sure to consult your medical professional.

General Headache Blend No. 1
- 4 drops Wintergreen
- 3 drops German Chamomile
- 2 drops Lavender
- 2 drops Copaiba
- 1 drop Clove

General Headache Blend No. 2
- 6 drops Peppermint
- 4 drops Eucalyptus Globulus
- 2 drops Myrrh

Recommendations:
Brain Power · Clarity · Clove
Copaiba · Deep Relief Roll-On
Dorado Azul
Eucalyptus Globulus
Lavender · M-Grain · Myrrh
PanAway · Peppermint
R.C. · Raven · Relieve It
Rosemary · Spearmint
Stress Away Roll-On
Tranquil Roll-On
Valerian · Wintergreen

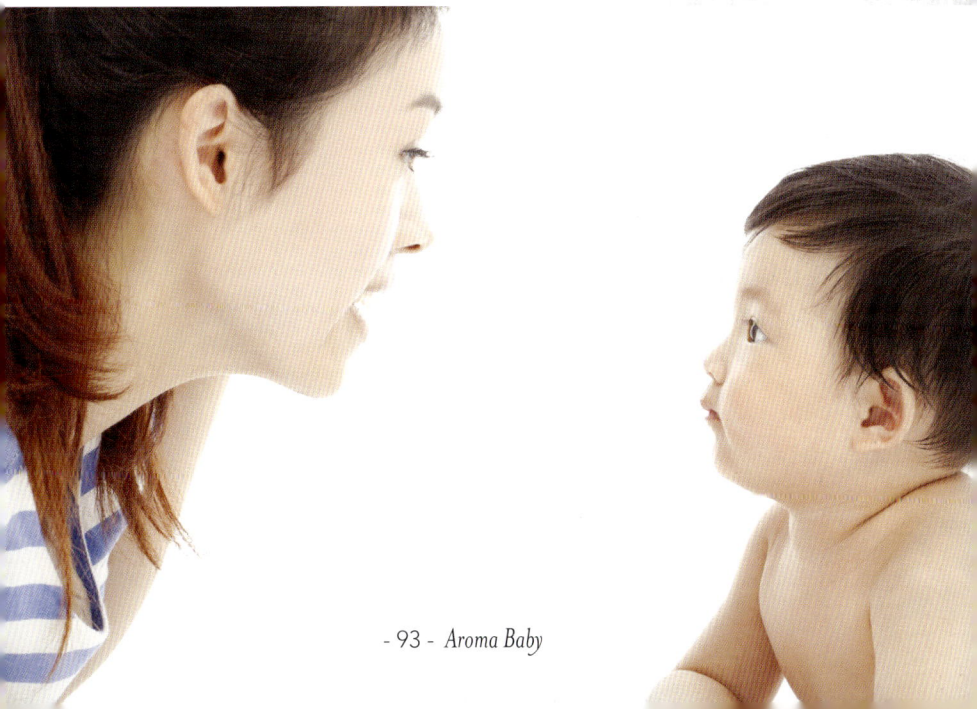

Inhalation:
- Diffuse your choice of oils for ½ hour every 4-6 hours or as desired.
- Put 2-3 drops of your chosen oil in your hands and rub them together, cup your hands over your nose, and inhale throughout the day as needed.
- Put 8-10 drops of oil on a cotton ball or tissue and put it in an air vent in your house, vehicle, hotel room, etc.
- If diffusing while sleeping, set your timer for the desired length of time for automatic shut off.

Topical:
- Dilute 50:50 and apply 1-3 drops on the back of the neck, behind the ears, on the temples, on the forehead, and under the nose. Be careful to keep away from eyes and eyelids.
- Massage 2-4 drops of oil neat on the soles of the feet just before bedtime.
- Place a warm compress with 1-2 drops of chosen oil on the back.

Ingestion & Oral:
- Take 1 capsule with desired oil 2 times daily.
- Place 1 drop on the tongue and then push it against the roof of the mouth.
- Put 2-3 drops of oil in a spoonful of Blue Agave, Yacon Syrup, maple syrup, coconut oil, milk, etc.
- Put the desired amount of oils in a glass of rice milk, almond milk, goat milk, carrot juice, NingXia Red, or even water and then drink it.

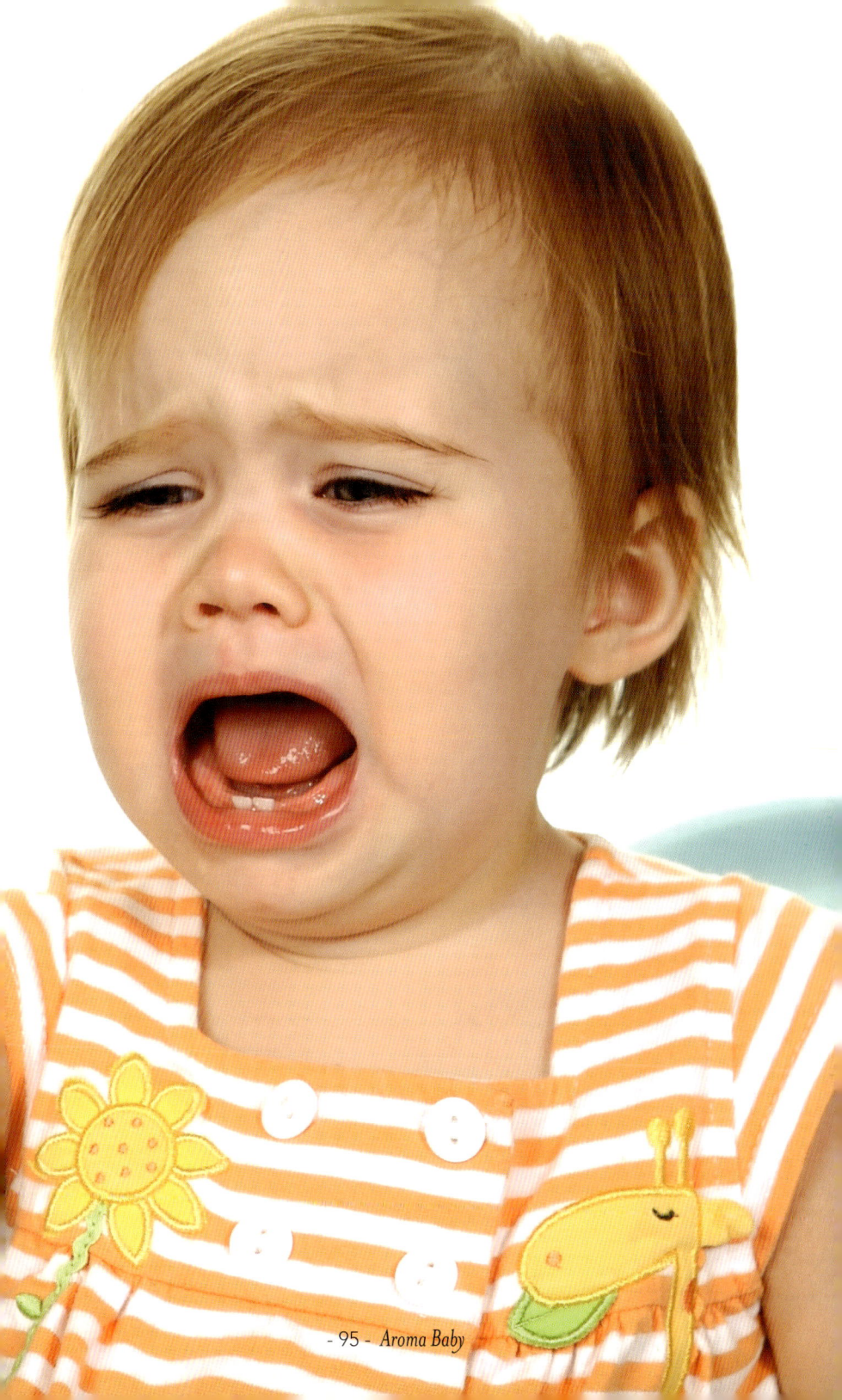

HEARTBURN

You may have never experienced heartburn until pregnancy. The progesterone levels slowing your digestive system will generally return to normal after delivery. Many heartburn remedies on the market are not recommended for women during pregnancy. Contrary to what you might think, lemon juice is actually one of the best remedies for heartburn. Though lemons have a degree of acid, they are actually alkaline-forming in the body. Squeeze half a lemon in 8 ounces of water and sip when you wake up each morning.

Lemon juice helps trigger the stomach to stop making digestive acids, and this action can help alleviate heartburn and other stomach issues.

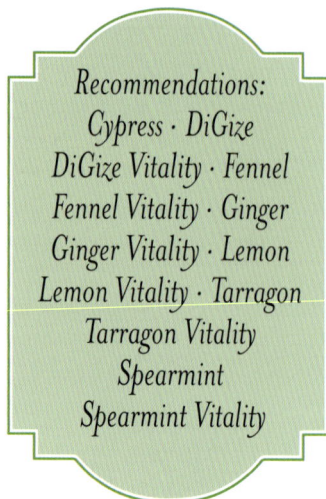

Recommendations:
Cypress · DiGize
DiGize Vitality · Fennel
Fennel Vitality · Ginger
Ginger Vitality · Lemon
Lemon Vitality · Tarragon
Tarragon Vitality
Spearmint
Spearmint Vitality

Inhalation:
- Diffuse your choice of oils for ½ hour every 4-6 hours or as desired.
- Put 2-3 drops of your chosen oil in your hands and rub them together, cup your hands over your nose, and inhale throughout the day as needed.
- Put 8-10 drops of oil on a cotton ball or tissue and put it in an air vent in your house, vehicle, hotel room, etc.
- If diffusing while sleeping, set your timer for the desired length of time for automatic shut off.

Topical:
- Apply 2-3 drops diluted 50:50 to stomach, abdomen, and throat.
- You may also apply 2-3 drops on the Vita Flex stomach point of the right foot.

Ingestion & Oral:
- Take 1 capsule with desired Vitality line oil 2 times daily.
- Put 2-3 drops of Vitality line oil in a spoonful of Blue Agave, Yacon Syrup, maple syrup, coconut oil, milk, etc.
- Put the desired amount of oils in a glass of rice milk, almond milk, goat milk, carrot juice, NingXia Red, or even water and then drink it.

HEMORRHOIDS

With the straining and slowing of the digestive system, many women report a temporary case of hemorrhoids during pregnancy, particularly toward the end when pressure from the uterus on the digestive tract is strongest. This condition may affect them for a short time after birth.

Recommendations:
Aroma Life · Aroma Siez
Cistus · Cypress
Deep Relief · Helichrysum
KidScents Tender Tush
Lemon · Melrose · Myrrh
PanAway · Peppermint
Purification · Rose Ointment
Spikenard

Tender Tush Blend No. 1
- 4 drops Basil
- 1 drop Cistus
- 1 drop Cypress
- 1 drop Helichrysum

Mix with Rose Ointment for dilution and easier application.

Tender Tush Blend No. 2
- 4 drops Myrrh
- 3 drops Cypress
- 2 drops Helichrysum

Mix with Rose Ointment for dilution and easier application.

Topical:
- Apply single oils or blends neat or diluted, depending on the oils that are used.
- Use a rectal implant (enema) of your choice with the above formulas by diluting with V6; place in rectum with a small syringe 1 time every other day for 6 days. It is best done at night to be able to retain as long as possible.
- Apply 3-5 drops diluted 50:50 on location. This may sting but usually brings relief with 1 or 2 applications.

Ingestion & Oral:
- Take 1 capsule with desired oil 2 times daily.
- Put 2-3 drops of oil in a spoonful of Blue Agave, Yacon Syrup, maple syrup, coconut oil, milk, etc.
- Put the desired amount of oils in a glass of rice milk, almond milk, goat milk, carrot juice, NingXia Red, or even water.

HIVES

As your belly begins to expand, this can cause itchiness, dryness, hives, and rashes. Most of these are mild, but 1-2% of women will develop the more serious skin condition, PUPP.

- Apply 2-4 drops diluted 50:50 on location as needed.
- Place a cold compress on location as needed.

Recommendations:
Eucalyptus Radiata
KidScents Tender Tush
Lavender · Myrrh
Peace & Calming · Peppermint
Ravintsara · Rose Ointment
RutaVaLa · RutaVaLa Roll-On
Stress Away Roll-On
Tea Tree (Melaleuca Alternifolia)
Tranquil Roll-On

INDIGESTION

During pregnancy, all sorts of foods become either extremely appetizing or the opposite. Sometimes you find you can't stomach the scent of certain foods. A combination of all three ways of using essential oils can help ease this during your term.

Recommendations:
Cedarwood · Frankincense
Frankincense Vitality · Ginger
Ginger Vitality · Harmony · Humility
Lavender · Lavender Vitality · Marjoram
Marjoram Vitality · Peace & Calming
Peppermint · Peppermint Vitality · Rose
RutaVaLa · RutaVaLa Roll-On
Sandalwood · Sacred Frankincense
Tranquil Roll-On · Trauma Life
Valerian · Valor · Valor Roll-On

Inhalation:
- Diffuse your choice of oils for ½ hour every 4-6 hours or as desired.
- Put 2-3 drops of your chosen oil in your hands and rub them together, cup your hands over your nose, and inhale throughout the day as needed.
- Put 8-10 drops of oil on a cotton ball or tissue and put it in an air vent in your house, vehicle, hotel room, etc.

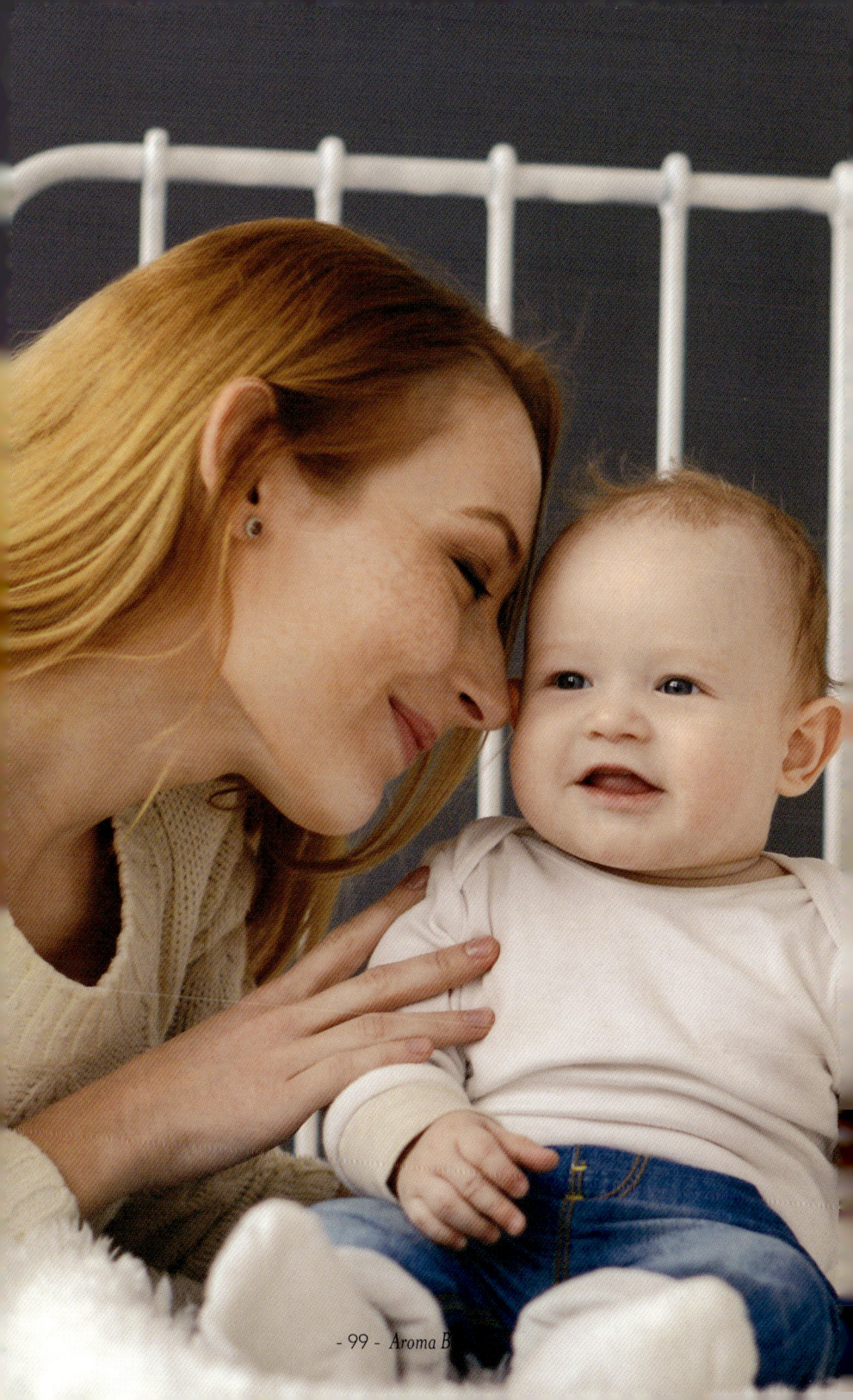

- If diffusing while sleeping, set your timer for the desired length of time for automatic shut off.

Topical:
- Apply any of the desired oils diluted 50:50 on temples, neck, and shoulders 2 times daily or as needed.
- Add desired oil to bath salts and incorporate into daily bathing.

Ingestion & Oral:
- Take 1 capsule with desired oil 2 times daily.
- Put 2-3 drops of oil in a spoonful of Blue Agave, Yacon Syrup, maple syrup, coconut oil, milk, etc.
- Put the desired amount of oils in a glass of rice milk, almond milk, goat milk, carrot juice, NingXia Red, or even water and then drink it.

INSECT BITES

Insect bites can cause more than just irritation. They can cause allergic reactions, infections and series dissease.

Stings and Bites Blend No. 1
- 10 drops Lavender
- 4 drops Eucalyptus Radiata
- 3 drops German Chamomile
- 2 drops Thyme

Spray sheets and clothing to kill any insects that might be imbedded in the cloth.

Recommendations:
Citronella · Copaiba ·Dorado Azul
Eucalyptus Radiata · Lavender
Lemongrass · Melrose
PanAway · Palo Santo · Peppermint
Purification · Rosemary
Tea Tree (Melaleuca Alternifolia)
Thieves

Insect Bite Blend No. 2
- 20 drops Palo Santo
- 20 drops Idaho Tansy
- 10 drops Eucalyptus Blue

Rub a small amount on skin or use in spray bottle.

Topical:
- Apply 1-2 drops of the sting and bite blends neat or diluted 50:50 on location 2-4 times daily.

INSECT REPELLENT

Preventing insect bites is really important during pregnancy. Mosquitoes can carry disease and this can pose a threat to your health and that of your baby.

Insect Repellent Blend No. 1
- 9 drops Idaho Tansy
- 6 drops Peppermint
- 6 drops Citronella

Insect Repellent Blend No. 2
- 6 drops Idaho Tansy
- 6 drops Palo Santo

Topical:
- Mix together and use undiluted or diluted with an ounce of distilled water.
- Apply 1-6 drops neat or diluted, depending on size of affected area, 3-5 times daily.

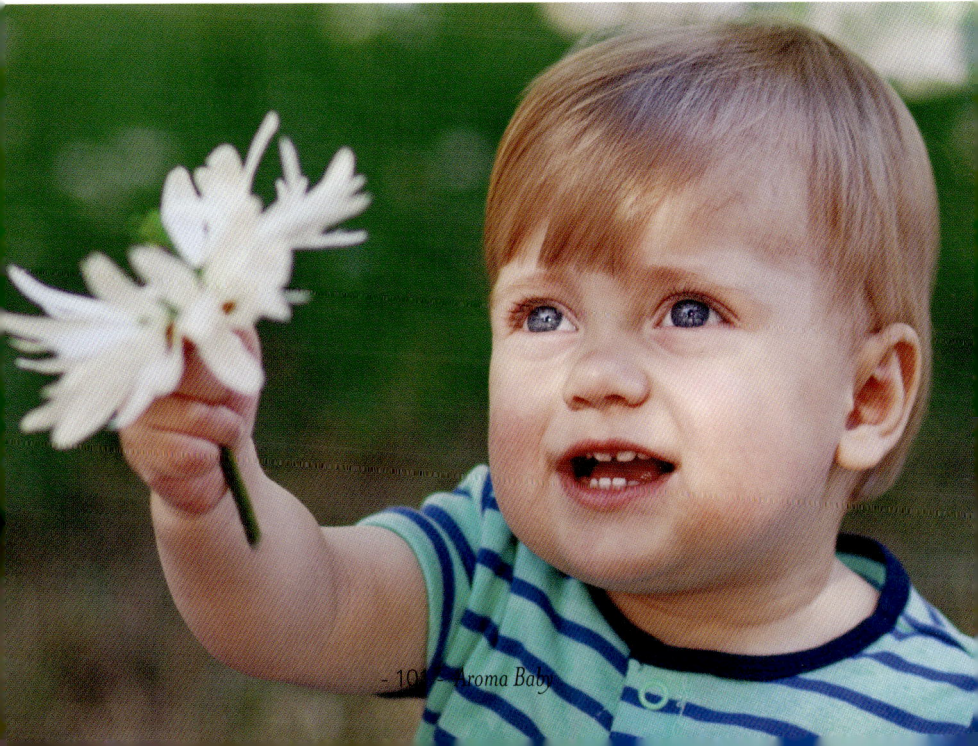

INSOMNIA

Melatonin production during pregnancy as well as other hormone changes and shifts in blood sugar can keep you from getting the sleep you need and deserve during pregnancy. Stress can only make this worse, and stressing about the whole situation can make insomnia infuriating. The important thing is to relax, get sleep at every opportunity, and use essential oils to boost your body's natural sleep cues.

Recommendations:
Cedarwood · Dream Catcher
Gentle Baby · Harmony,
Lavender · Orange, Peace & Calming
NingXia Red · OmegaGize3
Prenolone Plus Body Cream
Progessence Plus · RutaVaLa
RutaVaLa Roll-On · SleepEssence
Stress Away · Stress Away Roll-On
Valerian · Valor · Valor Roll-On
Tranquil Roll-On
Trauma Life

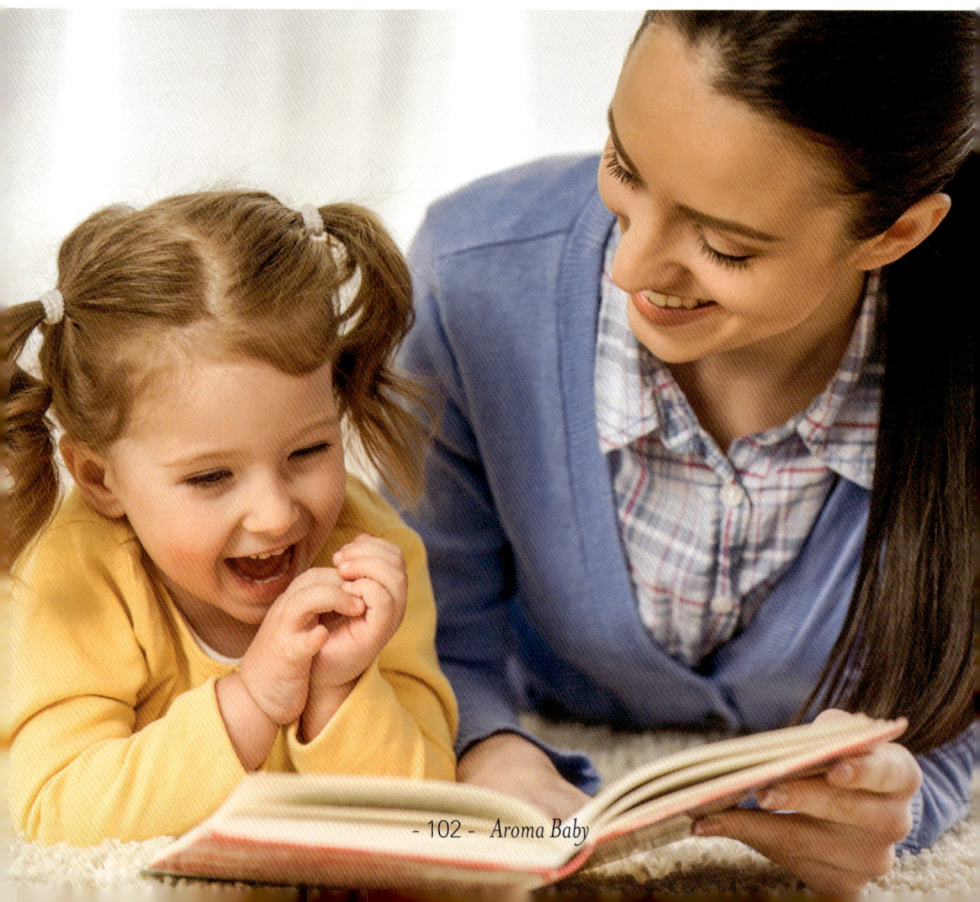

Insomnia Blend
- 12 drops Orange
- 8 drops Lavender
- 4 drops Dorado Azul
- 3 drops Valerian
- 2 drops Roman Chamomile

Inhalation:
- Diffuse 30-60 minutes at bedtime.
- Apply 1-3 drops on a cotton ball and place on or near your pillow.
- Put 2-3 drops of your chosen oil in your hands and rub them together, cup your hands over your nose, and inhale as needed.
- Put 8-10 drops of oil on a cotton ball or tissue and put it in an air vent in your house, vehicle, hotel room, etc.
- If diffusing while sleeping, set your timer for the desired length of time for automatic shut off.

Topical:
- Apply 1-3 drops neat to shoulders, stomach, and on bottoms of feet.
- Mix 6-8 drops of oils with ¼ cup Epsom salt or baking soda in hot water and add to hot bath water while tub is filling. Soak in bathtub for 20 to 30 minutes or until water cools.
- Rub 1-2 drops of oil on the temples and back of neck several times daily.
- Place a warm compress with 1-2 drops of chosen oil on the back.

Ingestion & Oral:
- Take 1 capsule with desired oil 2 times daily.
- Take 1 capsule of Lavender oil or any desired oil undiluted or diluted 50:50 1 hour before bedtime.
- Put 2-3 drops of oil in a spoonful of Blue Agave, Yacon Syrup, maple syrup, coconut oil, milk, etc.
- Put the desired amount of oils in a glass of rice milk, almond milk, goat milk, carrot juice, NingXia Red, or even water and then drink it.

ITCHING

Itching during pregnancy can often be due to dry skin and the expansion of skin tissue to accommodate the growth of your baby. It can also be a symptom of impaired liver function, insect bites, allergies, or overexposure to chemicals or sunlight.

> **Recommendations:**
> Aroma Siez · ClaraDerm · DiGize
> KidScents Tender Tush · LavaDerm
> Cooling Mist · Lavender · Melrose
> Nutmeg · Oregano · Patchouli
> Peppermint · Purification
> Regenolone Moisturizing Cream
> Rose Ointment
> Thieves · Vetiver

Topical:
- Apply 1-2 drops neat on location several times daily as needed.
- Dilute 50/50 and apply on location 3-6 times daily.
- Spray LavaDerm Cooling Mist or ClaraDerm if condition is evident on the skin.

KIDNEY PROBLEMS

As with all serious conditions, you should immediately consult a health care professional if you suspect a kidney infection or diminished kidney function of any kind.

> **Recommendations:**
> 3 Wise Men · Cistus
> Frankincense · Gentle Baby
> Geranium · Helichrysum, Juniper
> Lemongrass · Longevity · Melrose
> Myrrh · Purification · Rosemary
> Sacred Frankincense
> Thieves · Thyme

Inhalation:
- Diffuse your choice of oils for ½ hour every 4-6 hours or as desired.
- Put 2-3 drops of your chosen oil in your hands and rub them together, cup your hands over your nose, and inhale throughout the day as needed.
- Put 8-10 drops of oil on a cotton ball or tissue and put it in an air vent in your house, vehicle, hotel room, etc.

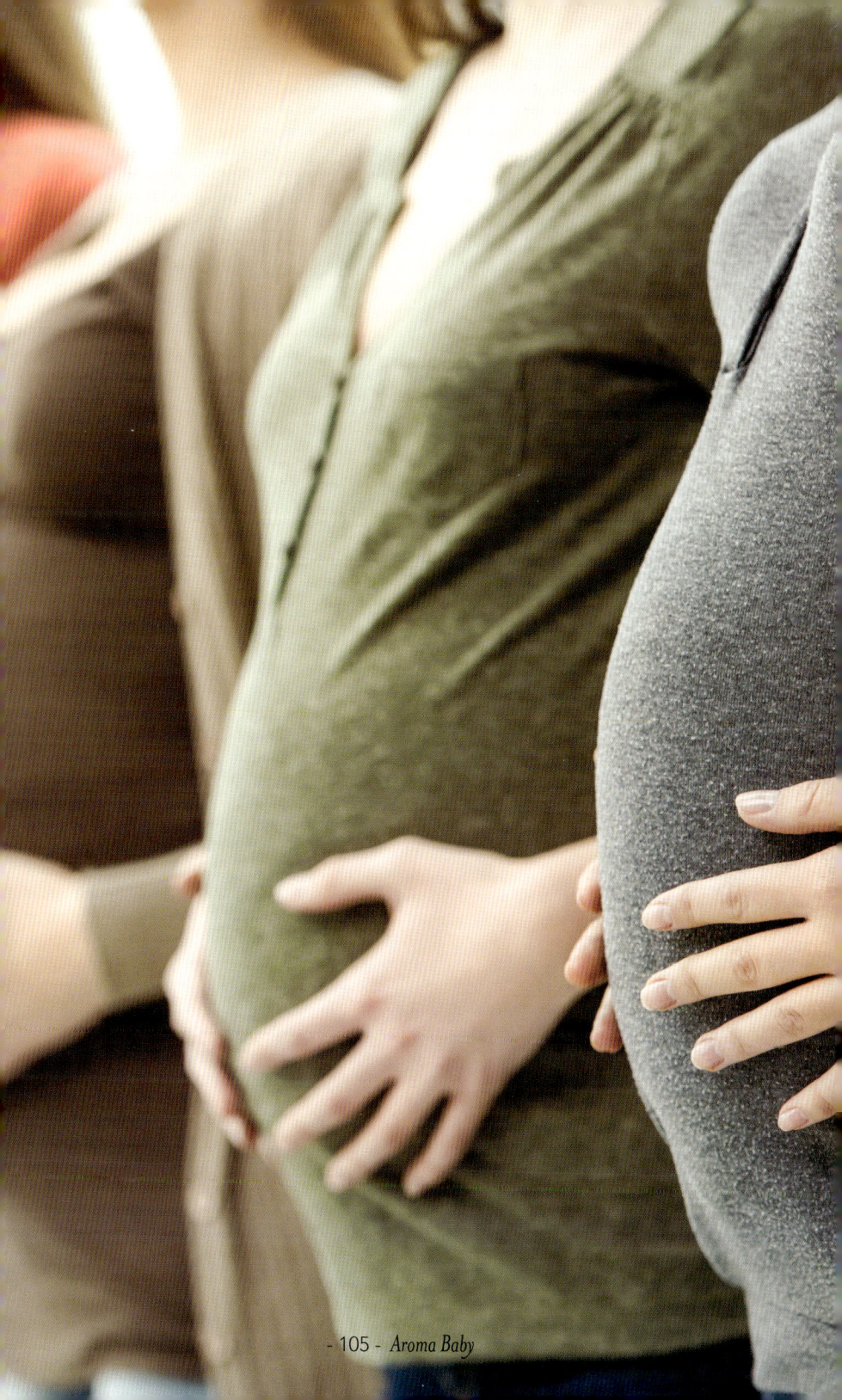

- If diffusing while sleeping, set your timer for the desired length of time for automatic shut off.

Topical:
- Massage 2-4 drops of oil neat on the soles of the feet Vita Flex points just before bedtime.
- Place a cold compress with 1-2 drops of chosen oil over the kidney area 1-2 times daily.

Ingestion & Oral:
- Take 2 capsules with desired oil 2 times daily for 10 days.
- Put 2-3 drops of oil in a spoonful of Blue Agave, Yacon Syrup, maple syrup, coconut oil, milk, etc.
- Put the desired amount of oils in a glass of rice milk, almond milk, goat milk, carrot juice, NingXia Red, or even water and then drink it.

LACTATION (BOOST)

Inhalation:
- Diffuse your choice of oils for ½ hour every 4-6 hours or as desired.
- Put 2-3 drops of your chosen oil in your hands and rub them together, cup your hands over your nose, and inhale throughout the day as needed.

Recommendations:
Fennel · Fennel Vitality
Joy · Myrrh
Stress Away

- Put 8-10 drops of oil on a cotton ball or tissue and put it in an air vent in your house, vehicle, hotel room, etc.
- If diffusing while sleeping, set your timer for the desired length of time for automatic shut off.

Topical:
- Apply 1-2 drops neat on location several times daily as needed, preferably after feeding.
- Dilute 50/50 and apply on location 3-6 times daily just after feeding.

Ingestion & Oral:

- Take 2 capsules with 1-2 drops Fennel Vitality 2 times daily for 10 days.
- Put 2-3 drops of Fennel Vitality in a spoonful of Blue Agave, Yacon Syrup, maple syrup, coconut oil, milk, etc. and take every 2 hours, preferably after feeding.
- If any family history of epilepsy or seizures exists, refrain from using Fennel or high ketone oils such as Basil, Rosemary, Sage, and Tansy oils. Use extra caution if you decide to use any of these.

LACTATION (CALMING OVERPRODUCTION)

Inhalation:

- Diffuse your choice of oils for ½ hour every 4-6 hours or as desired.
- Put 2-3 drops of your chosen oil in your hands and rub them together, cup your hands over your nose, and inhale throughout the day as needed.
- Put 8-10 drops of oil on a cotton ball or tissue and put it in an air vent in your house, vehicle, hotel room, etc.
- If diffusing while sleeping, set your timer for the desired length of time for automatic shut off.

> *Recommendations:*
> *Clary Sage*
> *Peppermint*

Topical:

- Apply 1-2 drops neat on location several times daily as needed, preferably after feeding.
- Dilute 50/50 and apply on location 3-6 times daily just after feeding.

Ingestion & Oral:

- Take 2 capsules with 2 times daily for 10 days.
- Put 2-3 drops of Fennel Vitality in a spoonful of Blue Agave, Yacon Syrup, maple syrup, coconut oil, milk, etc. and take every 2 hours, preferably after feeding.
- If family history of epilepsy or seizures exists, refrain from using Fennel or high ketone oils such as Basil, Rosemary, Sage, and Tansy oils. Use extra caution if you decide to use any of these.

LABOR

Once labor has begun, this Labor Blend can help support a healthy delivery. It's important only to use this blend during delivery, not any time beforehand:

Labor Blend
(Use only after labor has started.)
- 5 drops Ylang Ylang
  (or Amazonian Ylang Ylang)
- 4 drops Helichrysum
- 2 drops Fennel
- 2 drops Peppermint
- 2 drops Clary Sage

Recommendations:
Gentle Baby · Geranium
German Chamomile · Forgiveness
Grounding · Highest Potential
Joy · Lavender · Myrrh
Rose · Helichrysum · Neroli
Peace & Calming
Sacred Mountain · Sandalwood
Valor · Valor Roll-On
White Angelica · Ylang Ylang

Inhalation:
- Diffuse your choice of oils for ½ hour every 4-6 hours or as desired.
- Put 2-3 drops of your chosen oil in your hands and rub them together, cup your hands over your nose, and inhale throughout the day as needed.
- Put 8-10 drops of oil on a cotton ball or tissue and put it in an air vent in your house, vehicle, hotel room, etc.
- If diffusing while sleeping, set your timer for the desired length of time for automatic shut off.
- Diffuse Gentle Baby, Joy, or Valor to reduce stress before and after the birth. Expectant fathers will also find this helps to reduce anxiety during delivery.

Topical:
- Massage 2-4 drops Labor Blend from above diluted 50:50 on reproductive Vita Flex points on the sides of the ankles. Apply ONLY after labor has started.
- Massage 2-4 drops Labor Blend from above on lower stomach and lower back.

LUPUS

Medical professionals consider any lupus pregnancy to be high risk. Each of the three types of lupus will carry its own set of risks for complication. In general, women who have lupus pre-pregnancy have an increased risk of miscarriage, premature delivery, and preeclampsia, as well as heart problems in the baby. While the number of complications for these pregnancies is under 50%, this is still a considerable number. Many physicians recommend looking to conceive when your health is at its best and your lupus is fully under control. Talk with your medical professional about what is right for you, and be sure to keep her or him in the know.

Recommendations:
Basil · Basil Vitality
Eucalyptus Globulus
Lavender · Lavender Vitality
Myrrh · Nutmeg · Nutmeg Vitality
PanAway · R.C. · Thieves
Thieves Vitality · Thyme
Thyme Vitality · Valor
Valor Roll-On · Wintergreen

Lupus Blend
- 10 drops Lavender
- 4 drops Eucalyptus Globulus
- 3 drops Myrrh
- 3 drops Nutmeg

Bath Salts: Using lupus blend above, add 30 drops to ½ cup Epsom salt or baking soda and add to hot bath. Soak for 20-30 minutes or until water cools.

Vita Flex: Massage PanAway on bottoms of the feet and follow 2 hours later with a foot massage using Thieves.

Topical: Massage 10-15 drops Basil over liver and on feet 2-3 times daily.

Sulfurzyme: Take 1-2 tablespoons of powder or 5 capsules 1-2 times daily.

Essentialzyme: Take 2-6 tablets 2 times daily.

MultiGreens: Take 2-4 capsules 2 times daily.

Inhalation:

- Diffuse your choice of oils for ½ hour every 4-6 hours or as desired.
- Put 2-3 drops of your chosen oil in your hands and rub them together, cup your hands over your nose, and inhale throughout the day as needed.
- Put 8-10 drops of oil on a cotton ball or tissue and put it in an air vent in your house, vehicle, hotel room, etc.
- If diffusing while sleeping, set your timer for the desired length of time for automatic shut off.

Topical:

- Apply 1-2 drops neat on temples and back of neck as desired.
- Have Raindrop Technique 1-2 times weekly.
- Have body massage using desired essential oils once every other day.

Ingestion & Oral:

- Take 1 capsule with 5 drops of desired oil 2 times daily.
- Put 2-3 drops of oil in a spoonful of Blue Agave, Yacon Syrup, maple syrup, coconut oil, milk, etc.
- Put the desired amount of oils in a glass of rice milk, almond milk, goat milk, carrot juice, NingXia Red, or even water and then drink it.

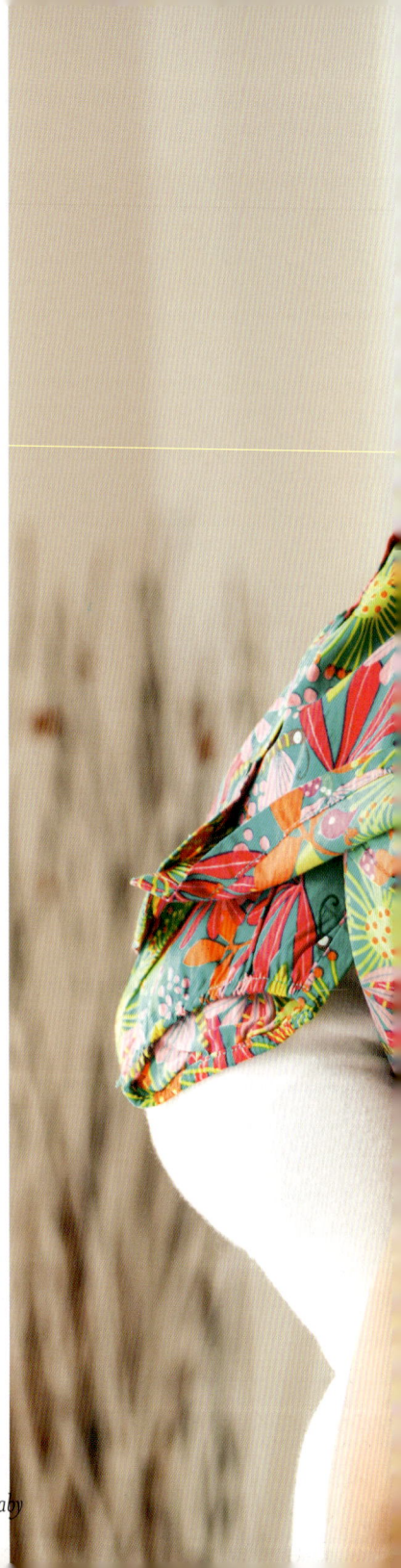

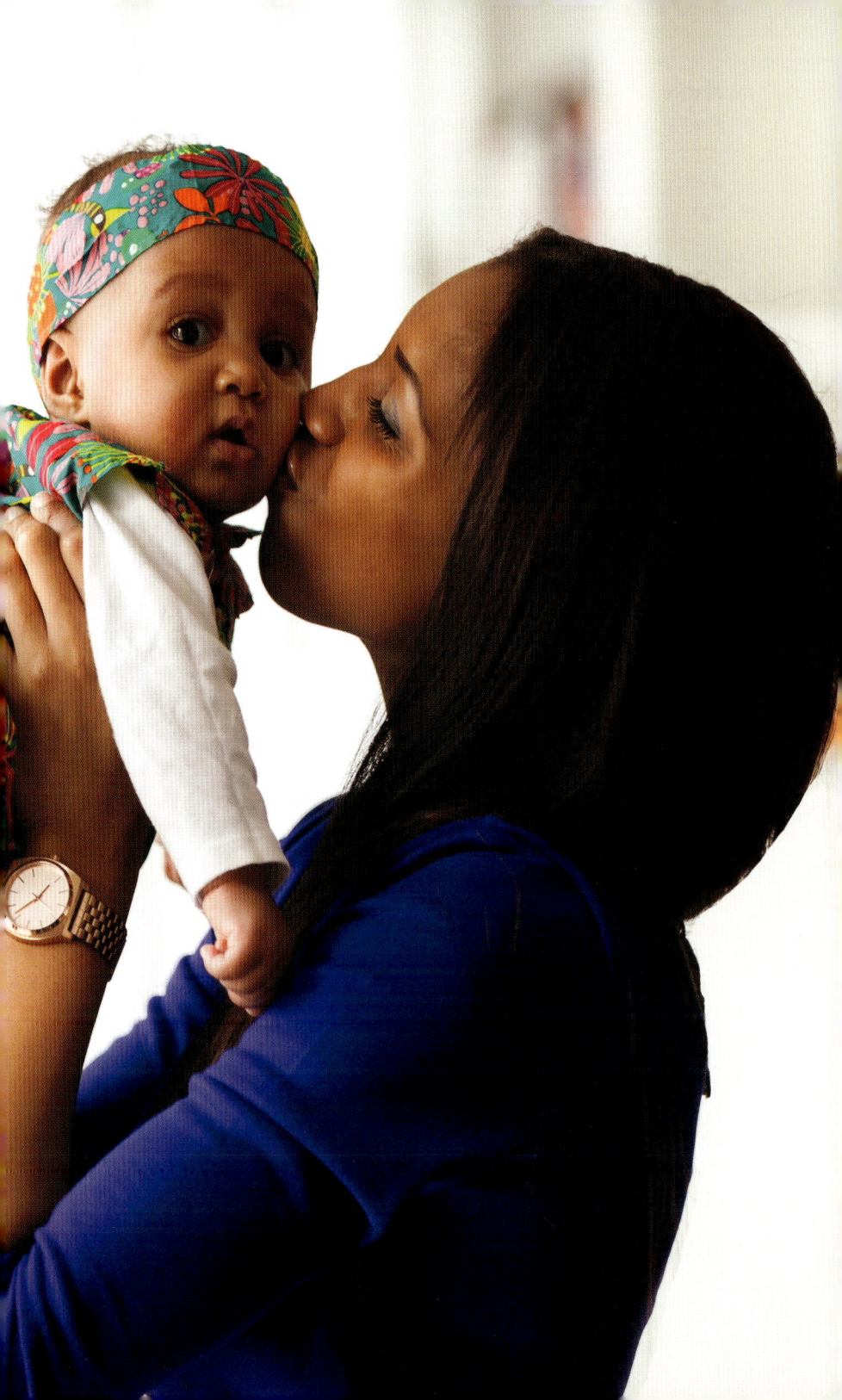

MIGRAINES

Like most headaches, migraines are usually caused by hormone shifts, circulatory problems, stress, sugar imbalance (hypoglycemia), structural (spinal) misalignments, and blood pressure—all of which can be issues during pregnancy. If you suspect an increase in blood pressure or blood sugar, be sure to consult your medical professional.

Recommendations:
Brain Power · Clarity · Clove
Copaiba · Deep Relief Roll-On
Dorado Azul · Eucalyptus Globulus
Lavender · M-Grain · Myrrh
PanAway · Peppermint · R.C.
Raven · Relieve It · Rosemary
Spearmint · Stress Away Roll-On
Tranquil Roll-On
Valerian · Wintergreen

General Headache Blend No. 1
- 4 drops Wintergreen
- 3 drops German Chamomile
- 2 drops Lavender
- 2 drops Copaiba
- 1 drop Clove

General Headache Blend No. 2
- 6 drops Peppermint
- 4 drops Eucalyptus Globulus
- 2 drops Myrrh

Inhalation:
- Diffuse your choice of oils for ½ hour every 4-6 hours or as desired.
- Put 2-3 drops of your chosen oil in your hands and rub them together, cup your hands over your nose, and inhale throughout the day as needed.
- Put 8-10 drops of oil on a cotton ball or tissue and put it in an air vent in your house, vehicle, hotel room, etc.
- If diffusing while sleeping, set your timer for the desired length of time for automatic shut off.

Topical:
- Dilute 50:50 and apply 1-3 drops on the back of the neck, behind the ears, on the temples, on the forehead, and under the nose. Be careful to keep away from eyes and eyelids.
- Massage 2-4 drops of oil neat on the soles of the feet just before bedtime.
- Place a warm compress with 1-2 drops of chosen oil on the back.

Ingestion & Oral:

- Take 1 capsule with desired oil 2 times daily.
- Place 1 drop on the tongue and then push it against the roof of the mouth.
- Put 2-3 drops of oil in a spoonful of Blue Agave, Yacon Syrup, maple syrup, coconut oil, milk, etc.
- Put the desired amount of oils in a glass of rice milk, almond milk, goat milk, carrot juice, NingXia Red, or even water and then drink it.

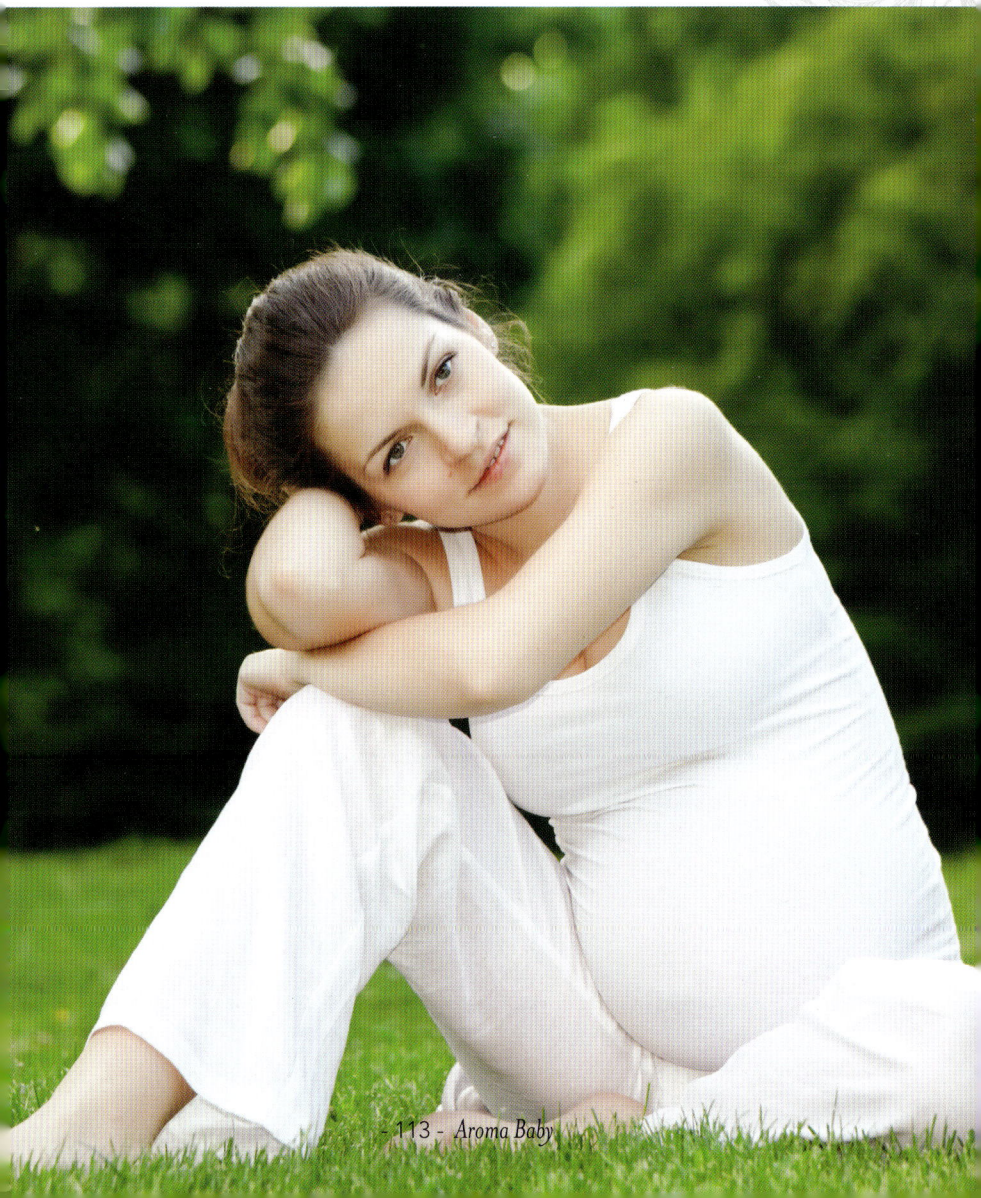

MORNING SICKNESS

Morning sickness is one of the first signs for many women that they are pregnant. It usually happens in the first trimester and tapers off in the 12th week, but some women report it throughout all times in their pregnancies. Despite the name, it can occur at any time of the day and is usually tied to your estrogen levels.

> **Recommendations:**
> Cedarwood · Frankincense
> Frankincense Vitality · Ginger
> Ginger Vitality · Harmony · Humility
> Lavender · Lavender Vitality · Marjoram
> Marjoram Vitality ·Peace & Calming
> Peppermint · Peppermint Vitality
> Rose · RutaVaLa · RutaVaLa Roll-On
> Sandalwood · Sacred Frankincense
> Tranquil Roll-On · Trauma Life
> Valerian · Valor · Valor Roll-On

Inhalation:

- Diffuse your choice of oils for ½ hour every 4-6 hours or as desired.
- Put 2-3 drops of your chosen oil in your hands and rub them together, cup your hands over your nose, and inhale throughout the day as needed.
- Put 8-10 drops of oil on a cotton ball or tissue and put it in an air vent in your house, vehicle, hotel room, etc.
- If diffusing while sleeping, set your timer for the desired length of time for automatic shut off.

Topical:

- Apply any of the desired oils diluted 50:50 on temples, neck, and shoulders 2 times daily or as needed.
- Add desired oil to bath salts and incorporate into daily bathing.

Ingestion & Oral:

- Take 1 capsule with desired oil 2 times daily.
- Put 2-3 drops of oil in a spoonful of Blue Agave, Yacon Syrup, maple syrup, coconut oil, milk, etc.
- Put the desired amount of oils in a glass of rice milk, almond milk, goat milk, carrot juice, NingXia Red, or even water and then drink it.

MUSCLE ACHES

Muscle aches and pains are a natural part of pregnancy. As your body expands and accommodates your baby, you'll find yourself using muscles you never knew you had. Unless the pain is severe, lingering, or causing distress, it should not pose a threat to your health or that of your baby. If, however, you experience unexplained bruising, changes in blood sugar, rash, fever, or sore throat, you should seek immediate medical attention.

Recommendations:
AromaSiez™ · Copaiba
Deep Relief™
Deep Relief Roll-On
Dorado Azul · Idaho Balsam Fir
Marjoram · PanAway™
Relieve It · Valor™
Wintergreen

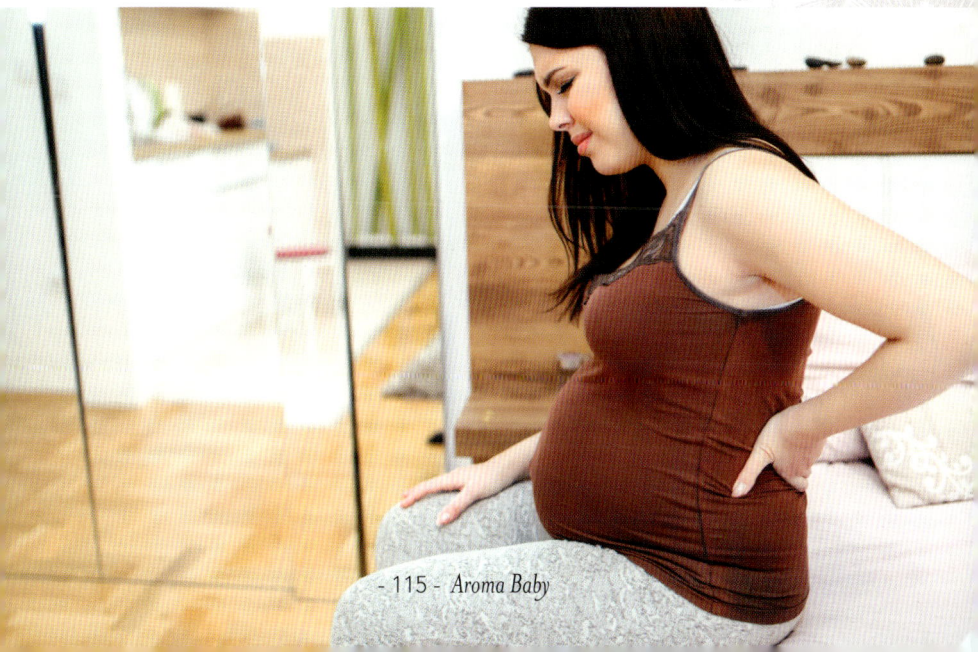

Muscle Relief Blend
- 5 drops Wintergreen
- 3 drops Lavender
- 3 drops Idaho Balsam Fir
- 2 drops Marjoram

Topical:
- Apply 2-4 drops neat on specific area 1-3 times daily or as needed.
- Apply 2-4 drops on Vita Flex area of foot.
- Use warm compress with 1-2 drops of chosen oil on the back daily.
- Apply Raindrop Technique 2 times weekly for 3 weeks.

NAILS (BRITTLE OR WEAK)

Poor or weak nails, often containing ridges, may indicate a sulfur, calcium, and/or Vitamin A deficiency. During pregnancy, most women report better growth, stronger nails, and better nail texture. But some women, who have great nails before pregnancy, experience weak, brittle, thin, cracked, and peeling nails. After delivery, however, hormonal changes will usually cause your nails to return to their pre-pregnancy texture and growth. Limit the use of nail polish and remover, your use of detergents, or excessive exposure to water.

Recommendations:
Citrus Fresh · DiGize
Frankincense
Idaho Balsam Fir
Lemon · Myrrh
Sacred Frankincense
Wintergreen

Nail Strengthening Blend
- 4 drops Wheat Germ Oil
- 2 drops Sacred Frankincense or Frankincense
- 2 drops Myrrh
- 2 drops Lemon
- 1 drop Wintergreen

Topical:
- Apply 1-3 drops neat on nails and at base of nails daily for 30 days.
- Apply 1 drop of the blend on each nail 2-3 times daily for 30 days.

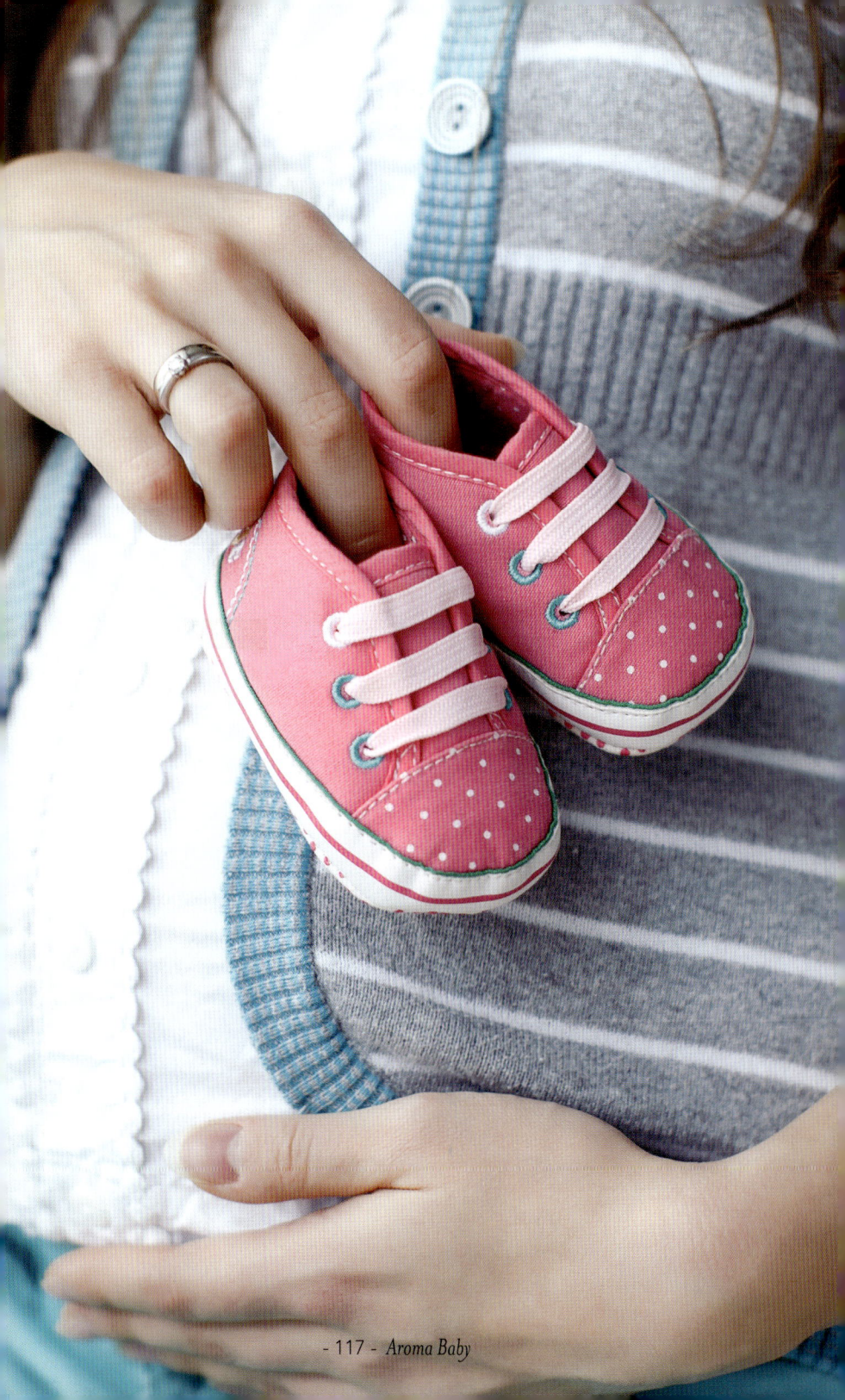

NAUSEA

The medical definition for "morning sickness" is "nausea and vomiting of pregnancy." Sometimes the symptoms are worse in the morning, but they can strike at any time; and for many women, they last all day long. The intensity varies from woman to woman.

Recommendations:
Cedarwood · Frankincense Frankincense Vitality · Ginger Ginger Vitality · Harmony · Humility Lavender · Lavender Vitality Marjoram · Marjoram Vitality · Peace & Calming Peppermint · Peppermint Vitality · Rose RutaVaLa · RutaVaLa Roll-On Sandalwood · Sacred Frankincense Tranquil Roll-On · Trauma Life Valerian · Valor · Valor Roll-On

Inhalation:

- Diffuse your choice of oils for ½ hour every 4-6 hours or as desired.
- Put 2-3 drops of your chosen oil in your hands and rub them together, cup your hands over your nose, and inhale throughout the day as needed.
- Put 8-10 drops of oil on a cotton ball or tissue and put it in an air vent in your house, vehicle, hotel room, etc.
- If diffusing while sleeping, set your timer for the desired length of time for automatic shut off.

Topical:

- Apply any of the desired oils diluted 50:50 on temples, neck, and shoulders 2 times daily or as needed.
- Add desired oil to bath salts and incorporate into daily bathing.

Ingestion & Oral:

- Take 1 capsule with desired oil 2 times daily.
- Put 2-3 drops of oil in a spoonful of Blue Agave, Yacon Syrup, maple syrup, coconut oil, milk, etc.
- Put the desired amount of oils in a glass of rice milk, almond milk, goat milk, carrot juice, NingXia Red, or even water and then drink it.

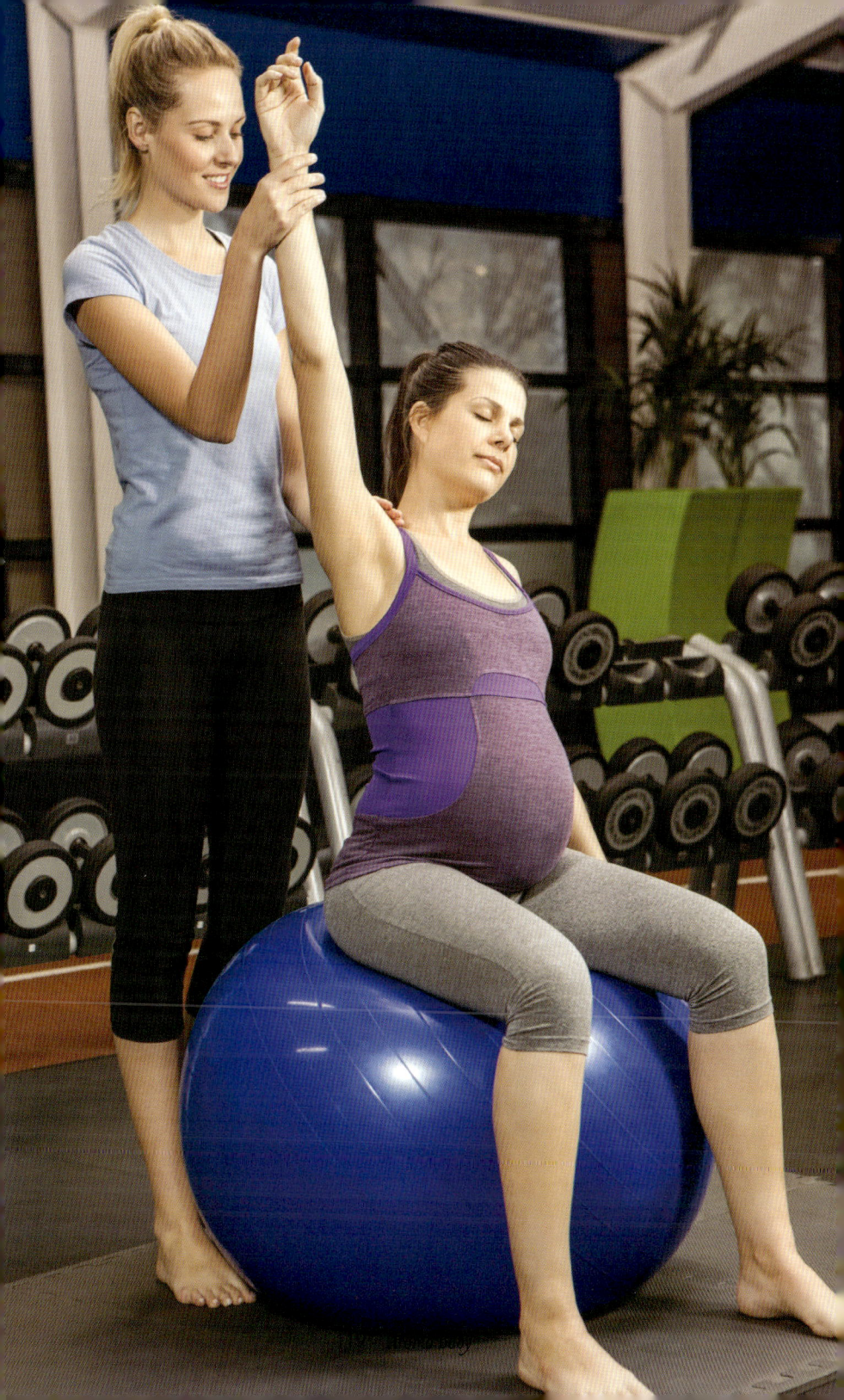

PERINEUM
(PREVENTING TEARS / EPISIOTOMY)

Oils like Lavender and Myrrh may help reduce stretch marks and improve the elasticity of the skin, helping to prevent tears. Geranium and Gentle Baby have similar effects and can be massaged on the perineum (tissue between vagina and rectum) to lower the risk of tearing during labor or the need for an episiotomy (an incision in the perineum) during birth.

> *Recommendations:*
> *ClaraDerm · Forgiveness*
> *Gentle Baby · Geranium*
> *Grounding · Helichrysum*
> *Highest Potential · Joy · Lavender*
> *Myrrh · Neroli · Peace & Calming*
> *Rose · Sacred Mountain*
> *Sandalwood · Tender Tush · Valor*
> *Valor Roll-On*
> *White Angelica*

Labor Blend
(Use only after labor has started.)
- 5 drops Ylang Ylang
  (or Amazonian Ylang Ylang)
- 4 drops Helichrysum
- 2 drops Fennel
- 2 drops Peppermint
- 2 drops Clary Sage

Inhalation:

- Diffuse your choice of oils for ½ hour every 4-6 hours or as desired.
- Put 2-3 drops of your chosen oil in your hands and rub them together, cup your hands over your nose, and inhale throughout the day as needed.
- Put 8-10 drops of oil on a cotton ball or tissue and put it in an air vent in your house, vehicle, hotel room, etc.
- If diffusing while sleeping, set your timer for the desired length of time for automatic shut off.
- Diffuse Gentle Baby, Joy, or Valor to reduce stress before and after the birth. Expectant fathers will also find this helps to reduce anxiety during delivery.

Topical:

- Massage 2-4 drops Labor Blend from above diluted 50:50 on reproductive Vita Flex points on the sides of the ankles. Apply ONLY after labor has started.
- Massage 2-4 drops Labor Blend from above on lower stomach and lower back.

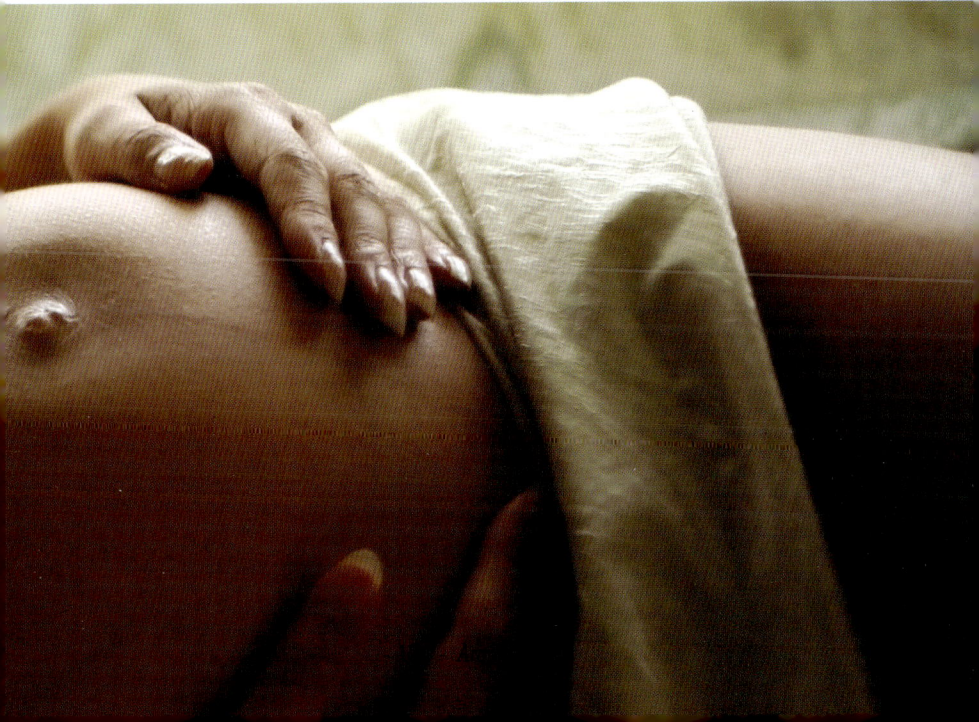

POISON IVY / OAK / SUMAC

Poison ivy, poison oak, and poison sumac are plants that contain an irritating, oily sap called urushiol, which triggers an allergic reaction when it comes into contact with skin. An itchy rash can appear within hours of exposure or several days later and usually develops into oozing blisters. Essential oils may be useful in avoiding corticosteroid shots for the inflammation.

Recommendations:
Basil · ClaraDerm · Gentle Baby
Geranium · KidScents Tender Tush
LavaDerm Cooling Mist · Lavender
Lemon · Melrose · Myrrh · Patchouli
Peppermint · Purification · R.C.
Rose · Rose Ointment · Rosemary
Sandalwood Moisture Cream
Spikenard
Tea Tree (Melaleuca Alternifolia)
Thieves Spray · Vetiver

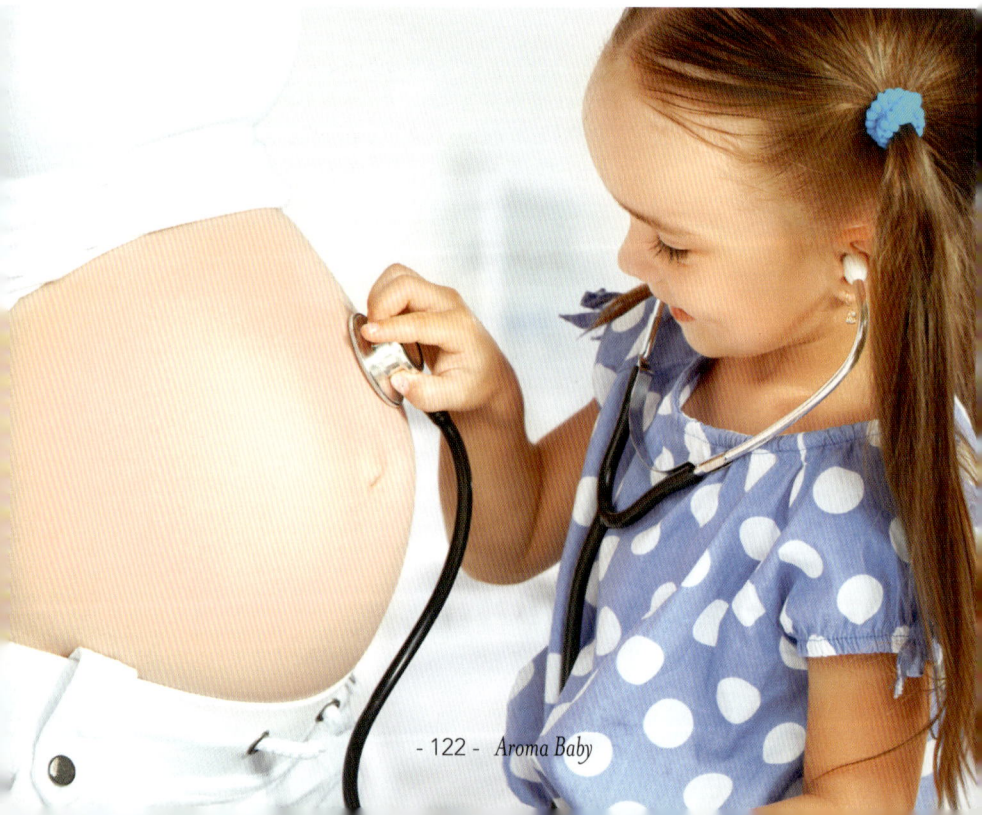

Topical:
- Apply 4-6 drops of oil diluted 50:50 to affected areas 2 times daily.
- Apply a cold compress on affected area 2 times daily.

POSTPARTUM DEPRESSION

"Baby blues" are normal for a few days after childbirth. Postpartum depression can follow and feel like more of the same or feel worse than before. It can also happen months after childbirth or pregnancy loss.

Recommendations:
Cedarwood · Clary Sage ·Dragon Time Frankincense · Hope · Joy · Lemon Melissa · Ocotea · Peace & Calming Prenolone Plus Body Cream Progessence Plus · RutaVaLa RutaVaLa Roll-On · Sandalwood Sacred Frankincense · Transformation Trauma Life

Inhalation:
- Diffuse recommended oils for 20 minutes 3 times daily.
- Put 2-3 drops of recommended oil in your hands and rub them together, cup your hands over your nose, and inhale 4-6 times daily.
- Put 8-10 drops of oil on a cotton ball or tissue and put it in an air vent in your house, vehicle, hotel room, etc.
- If diffusing while sleeping, set your timer for the desired length of time for automatic shut off.

Topical:
- Apply 2-4 drops neat on temples and back of neck 2-4 times daily or as needed.
- Applying a single drop under the nose is helpful and refreshing.
- Place a warm compress with 1-2 drops of chosen oil on the back.

Ingestion & Oral:
- Take 1 capsule with desired Vitality line oil 2 times daily.
- Put 2-3 drops of Vitality line oil in a spoonful of Blue Agave, Yacon Syrup, maple syrup, coconut oil, milk, etc.
- Put the desired amount of oils in a glass of rice milk, almond milk, goat milk, carrot juice, NingXia Red, or even water and then drink it.

PRE-ECLAMPSIA

Hypertension (high blood pressure above 140/90) can be a serious threat to pregnancy and result in dire complications. If high blood pressure continues after 20 weeks, it can develop into pre-eclampsia. Pre-eclampsia results in high levels of protein in the urine. If left untreated, pre-eclampsia may progress into eclampsia, characterized by seizures. Many medications can cause problems in pregnant women, so essential oils may provide a safe and natural alternative. Always consult your medical professional if you suspect or know you have high blood pressure during pregnancy. Most prenatal screenings will look for proteins and blood pressure that would imply pre-eclampsia.

Recommendations:
Aroma Life™ · Bergamot
Clary Sage · Frankincense
Jasmine · Lavender
NingXia Red · Ylang Ylang

Inhalation:
- Diffuse your choice of oils for ½ hour 3 times daily.
- Inhalation of Jasmine reduces anxiety in some people and may help to lower blood pressure.
- Put 2-3 drops of your chosen oil in your hands and rub them together, cup your hands over your nose, and inhale throughout the day as needed.
- Put 8-10 drops of oil on a cotton ball or tissue and put it in an air vent in your house, vehicle, hotel room, etc.
- If diffusing while sleeping, set your timer for the desired length of time for automatic shut off.

Topical:
- Apply 1-3 drops oil diluted 20:80 for a full body massage daily.
- Rub 1-2 drops of oil on the temples and back of neck several times daily.
- Place a warm compress with 1-2 drops of chosen oil on the back.
- For 3 minutes, massage 1-2 drops each of Aroma Life and Ylang Ylang (or Amazonian Ylang Ylang) on the heart Vita Flex point and over the heart and carotid arteries along the neck.
- Notice how the blood pressure will begin to drop within 5-20 minutes. Monitor the pressure and reapply as desired.

Ingestion & Oral:

- NingXia Red can be a great help for stabilizing blood pressure, particularly when taken regularly.
- Consider increasing your intake of magnesium, which acts as a smooth-muscle relaxant and as a natural calcium channel blocker for the heart, lowering blood pressure and dilating the heart blood vessels.

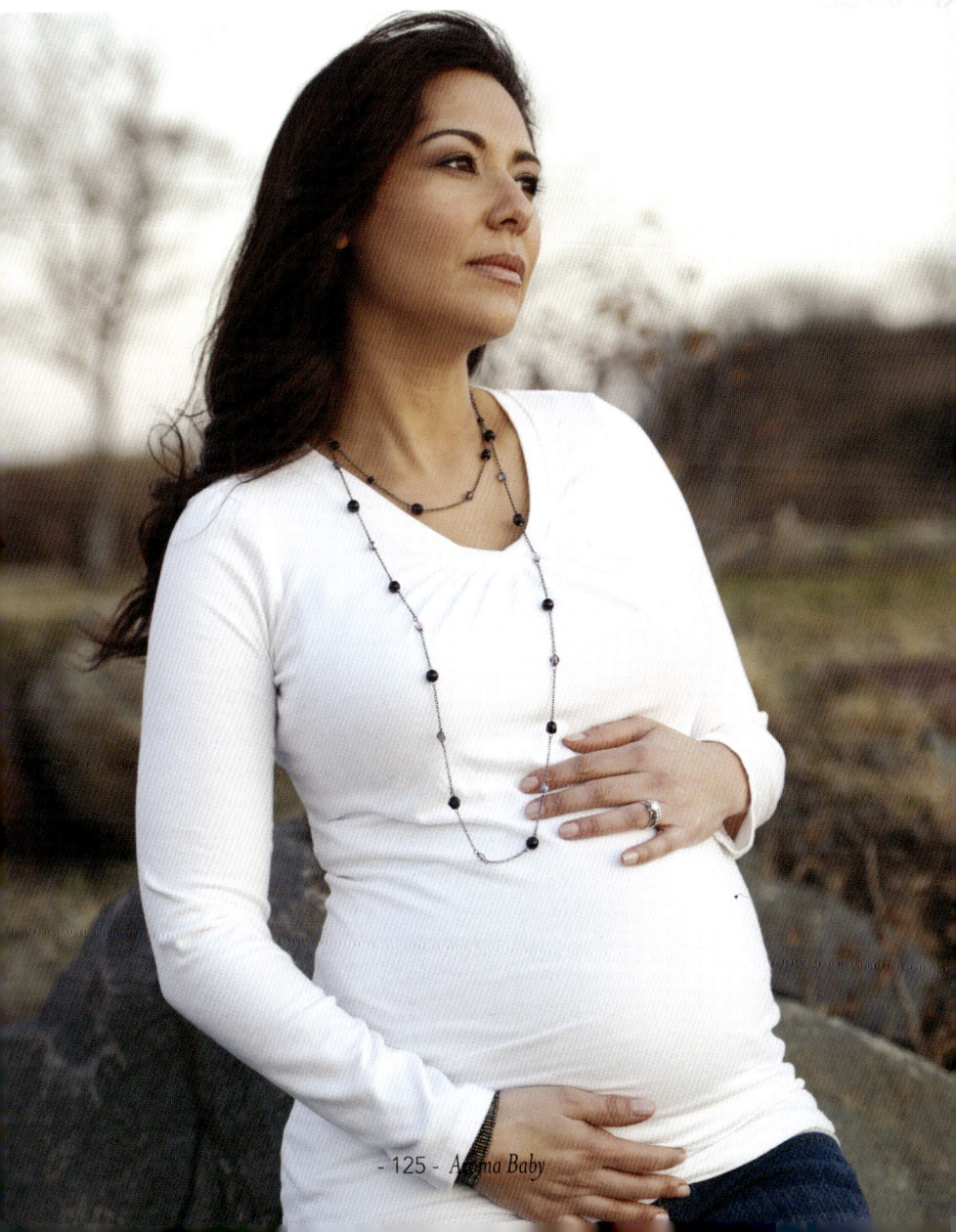

DIASTASIS SYMPHYSIS PUBIS
(PUBIS DIASTASIS / DSP)

This is an abnormally wide gap between the pubic bones, very near to a dislocation, without a fracture. This may happen during pregnancy or postpartum. The joint widening may expand from 4-5 mm to 9mm. This can cause pain and discomfort.

Recommendations:
Aroma Siez · Basil · Copaiba Helichrysum · Idaho Blue Spruce PanAway · Peppermint · Nutmeg Relieve It · Rosemary · Tarragon Thyme · Vetiver

Topical:

- Apply 6-10 drops diluted 50:50 on location 2 times daily or as needed.
- Place a warm compress on affected area 1-2 times daily; cold compress if inflamed.
- Massage 2-3 drops into Vita Flex points of the feet 2-4 times daily

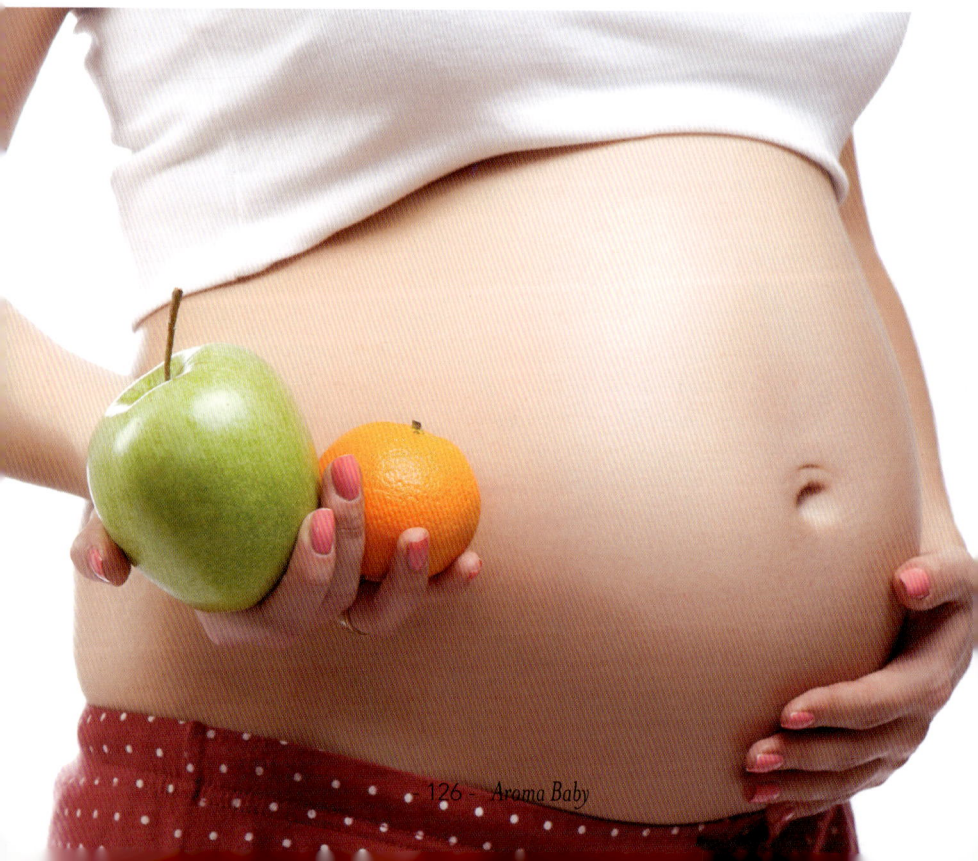

RESPIRATORY TRACT INFECTION

Essential oil blends work especially well in respiratory applications. Talk with your doctor if you have fever, pain, or sore throat.

Recommendations:
Copaiba · Bay · Laurel
Breathe Again Roll-On · Clove
Dorado Azul · Eucalyptus Blue
Eucalyptus Globulus
Eucalyptus Radiata · Exodus II
Idaho Balsam Fir · Idaho Ponderosa Pine
Lavender · Melaleuca Alternifolia
Melrose · Myrtle · Oregano · Palo Santo
PanAway · Pine · Purification · Raven
Ravintsara · R.C. · Rosemary · Thieves
Thieves Fresh Essence Plus Mouthwash
Thyme · Wintergreen

Respiratory Blend No. 1
- 6 drops Ravintsara
- 5 drops Clove
- 4 drops Myrrh
- 2 drops Palo Santo

Respiratory Blend No. 2
- 10 drops Dorado Azul
- 6 drops Eucalyptus Blue
- 5 drops Lavender
- 3 drops Eucalyptus Globulus

Inhalation:
- Diffuse your choice of oils, alternating between singles and blends, for ½ hour every 4-6 hours or as desired.
- Put 2-3 drops of your chosen oil in your hands and rub them together, cup your hands over your nose, and inhale throughout the day as needed.
- Put 8-10 drops of oil on a cotton ball or tissue and put it in an air vent in your house, vehicle, hotel room, etc.
- If diffusing while sleeping, set your timer for the desired length of time for automatic shut off.
- Add a few drops of oil to a bowl of boiling water. Position the face above the bowl and drape a towel over the head to create a vaporizing effect. Repeat 2-3 times daily.

Topical:
- Apply 2-6 drops neat or diluted 50:50 to the neck and chest as needed.
- Massage 2-3 drops on the lung Vita Flex points of the feet 2-4 times daily.
- Place a warm compress with 1-2 drops of chosen oil on the neck, chest, and upper back areas 1-3 times daily.

Ingestion & Oral:
- Take 1 capsule with desired oil 2 times daily.
- Put 2-3 drops of oil in a spoonful of Blue Agave, Yacon Syrup, maple syrup, coconut oil, milk, etc.
- Put the desired amount of oils in a glass of rice milk, almond milk, goat milk, carrot juice, NingXia Red, or even water and then drink it.
- Gargle a mixture of essential oils and water 4-8 times daily.

RESTLESS LEGS SYNDROME

(Willis-Ekbom disease) is a neurological disorder characterized by an irresistible urge to move the body to stop odd, irritating, or uncomfortable sensations such as crawling, tingling, itching, pulling, or burning. It commonly affects the legs but can also affect the torso, arms, and even phantom limbs. Around 16% of women report the sensation during pregnancy. It can be caused by low iron levels, particularly ferritin.

Recommendations:
Aroma Siez · Basil · Cypress
Lavender · Marjoram
Peace & Calming · RutaVaLa
RutaVaLa Roll-On
Stress Away Roll-On
Tranquil Roll-On
Valerian · Valor
Valor Roll-On

Inhalation:
- Diffuse your choice of oils for 20 minutes 4 times daily.
- Put 2-3 drops of your chosen oil in your hands and rub them together, cup your hands over your nose, and inhale throughout the day as needed.
- Put 8-10 drops of oil on a cotton ball or tissue and put it in an air vent in your house, vehicle, hotel room, etc.
- If diffusing while sleeping, set your timer for the desired length of time for automatic shut off.

Topical:
- Apply 2-4 drops neat as desired.
- Massage 2-4 drops of oil on the Vita Flex points of the feet before retiring.

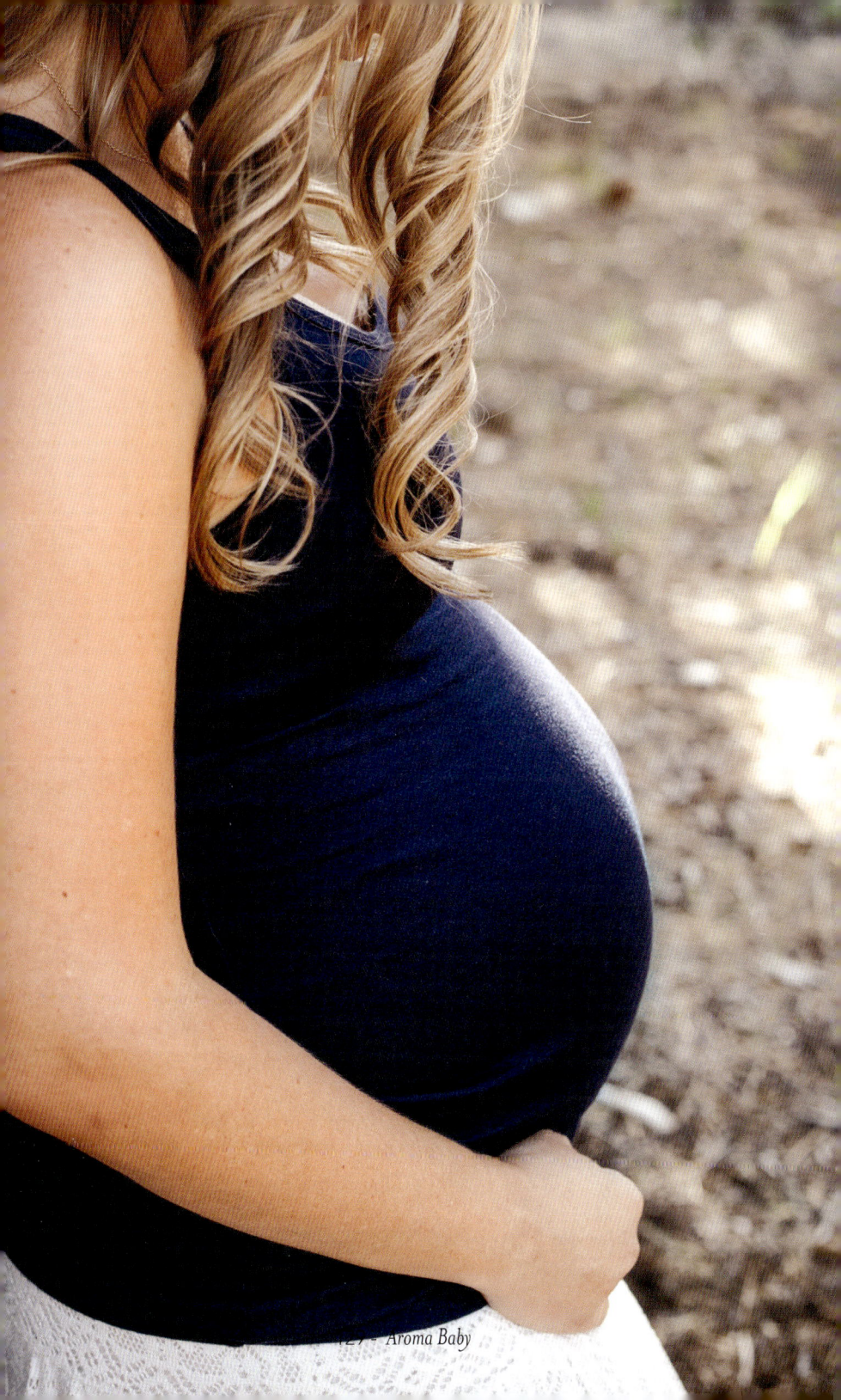

SKIN CARE

Bruise and Scrape Blend
(May be used on infants and children)
- 4 drops Lavender
- 1 drop Cistus
- 1 drop Myrrh

Infected Cut Blend
- 7 drops Geranium
- 5 drops Myrrh
- 3 drops   Melaleuca Alternifolia

Topical:
- Dilute recommended oils 50:50 and apply 2-6 drops on location 1-4 times daily.
- Apply LavaDerm Cooling Mist to the affected area.

Recommendations:
Cistus · Cypress · Frankincense
Helichrysym · Geranium
LavaDerm Cooling Mist
Lavender · Lemon · Melrose
Mountain Savory · Myrrh
Orange · Peace & Calming
Peppermint · Purification
Rose · Spikenard
Tea Tree (Melaleuca Alternifolia)
Tangerine
Tranquil Roll-On

Note: Peppermint can be helpful in treating wounds but may sting when applied to an open wound. To reduce discomfort, dilute with Lavender or mix in a sealing ointment before applying. When applied to a wound or cut that has a scab, a diluted Peppermint blend will soothe, cool, and reduce inflammation in damaged tissue.

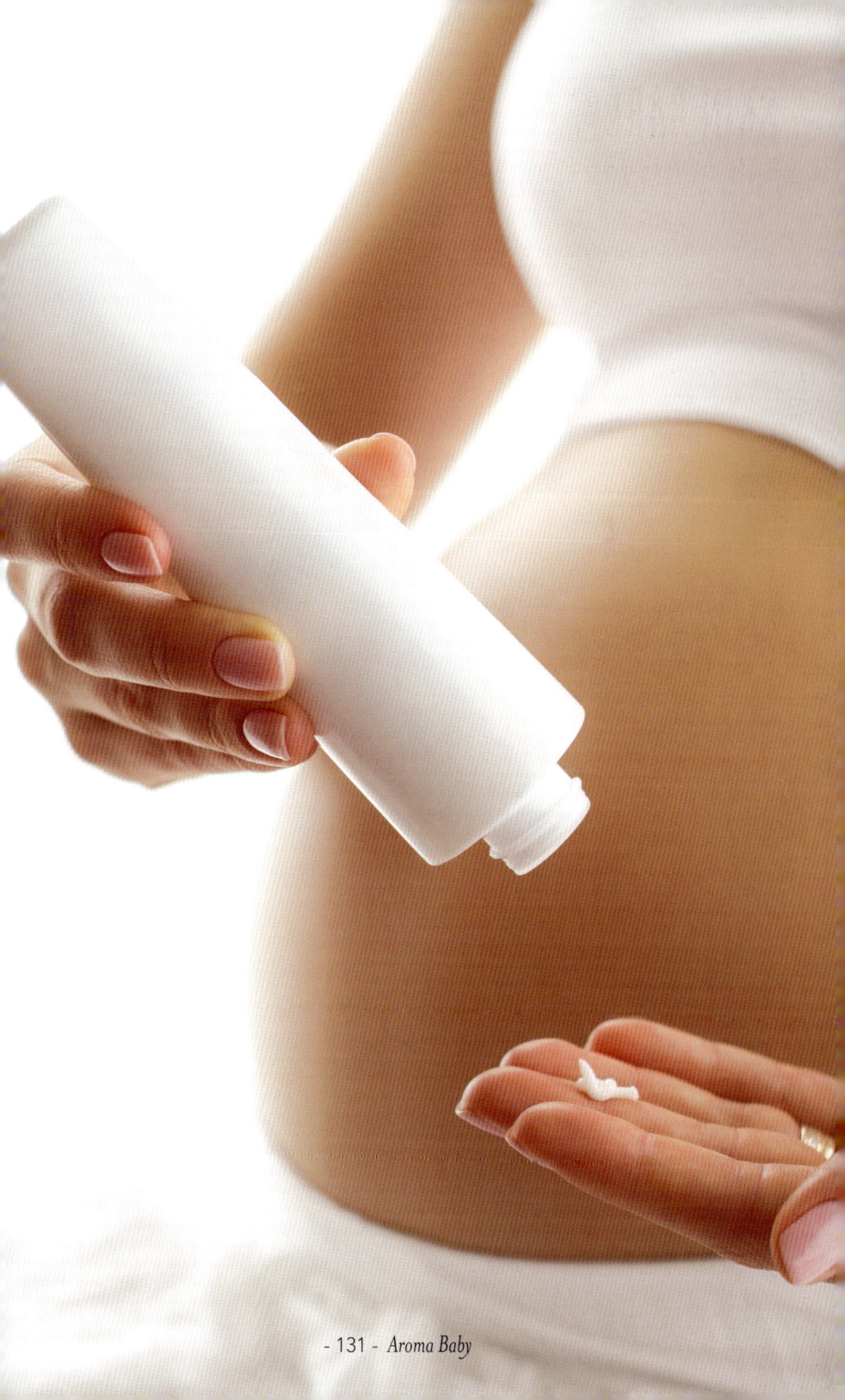

SORE NIPPLES
(DRY, CRACKED, ACHING)

One of the best ways to avoid infection and to be sure that breastfeeding is a rewarding experience for both mother and newborn is to take good care of your breasts, particularly your nipples.

> **Recommendations:**
> *Lavender · Myrrh · Melissa Patchouli · Rosemary Tea Tree (Melaleuca Alternifolia) Thyme*

Topical:
Dilute any of the above oils 20:80 and massage over breasts (avoiding the nipples) and on Vita Flex points of the feet. The same is true for the following blends:

Breast Blend No. 1
- 3 drops Thyme
- 7 drops PanAway
- 1 teaspoon V-6 Vegetable Oil Complex

Breast Blend No. 2
- 3 drops Lemon
- 4 drops Thyme
- 2 drops Melissa
- 1 teaspoon V-6 Vegetable Oil Complex

STRETCH MARKS

Stretch marks are most commonly associated with pregnancy but can also occur during growth spurts and periods of weight gain.

> **Recommendations:**
> *Elemi · Frankincense · Gentle Baby Geranium · KidScents Tender Tush Lavender · Myrrh · Rose Ointment Sacred Frankincense · Sensation Spikenard · Valor · White Angelica*

Topical:
- Apply 3-6 drops of oil neat or diluted 50:50 2 times daily.

THRUSH

This is a fungal mouth and throat infection, known for its creamy, curd-like patches in the oral cavity. Even though you contract thrush in the mouth, it can be a sign of systemic fungal overgrowth throughout your body. Thrush can usually be treated locally through the use of antifungal essential oils such as Clove, Cinnamon, Rosemary, Peppermint, and Rosewood.

Recommendations:
Cinnamon Bark
Cinnamon Bark Vitality · Clove
Clove Vitality · Geranium
Inner Defense · Lavender
Lavender Vitality · Melrose · Orange
Orange Vitality · Peppermint
Peppermint Vitality · Purification
Rosemary · Rosemary Vitality
Rosewood · Thieves
Thieves Lozenges (Hard/Soft)
Thieves Fresh Essence Plus Mouthwash
Thieves Spray · Thieves Vitality

Inhalation:
- Diffuse your choice of oils for ½ hour every 4-6 hours or as desired.
- Put 2-3 drops of your chosen oil in your hands and rub them together, cup your hands over your nose, and inhale throughout the day as needed.
- Put 8-10 drops of oil on a cotton ball or tissue and put it in an air vent in your house, vehicle, hotel room, etc.
- If diffusing while sleeping, set your timer for the desired length of time for automatic shut off.

Topical:
- Dilute 50:50 or 20:80 as needed and massage 3-4 drops on thymus (at clavicle notch, center of collarbone at base of throat) to stimulate the immune system. Also apply 3-6 drops on bottoms of the feet and on the chest. Also apply 5-10 drops on stomach. Do these applications 2 times daily.
- Massage 2-4 drops on relevant Vita Flex points on feet 2-4 times daily.

Ingestion & Oral:
- Take 1 capsule with desired oil 2-3 times daily between meals.
- Put 2-3 drops of oil in a spoonful of Blue Agave, Yacon Syrup, maple syrup, coconut oil, milk, etc.
- Put the desired amount of oils in a glass of rice milk, almond milk, goat milk, carrot juice, NingXia Red, or even water and then drink it.

- Gargle 3-5 times daily with Thieves Fresh Essence Plus Mouthwash.

Blend for Combating Gum Bleeding
- 2 drops Myrrh
- 2 drops Helichrysum
- 1 drop Thieves
- 1 drop Sacred Frankincense or Frankincense

Topical:
- Apply 1-2 drops diluted 50:50 on gums 2-3 times daily.

Ingestion & Oral:
- Take 1 capsule with desired oil 2 times daily.
- Put 2-3 drops of oil in a spoonful of Blue Agave, Yacon Syrup, maple syrup, coconut oil, milk, etc.
- Put the desired amount of oils in a glass of rice milk, almond milk, goat milk, carrot juice, NingXia Red, or even water and then drink it.
- Gargle 3-10 times daily with Thieves Fresh Essence Plus Mouthwash or as needed.
- Brush teeth and gums after every meal with Thieves AromaBright Toothpaste.

THYROID

Thyroid problems can be a challenge to your metabolism, especially as you bounce back from pregnancy. If you suspect thyroid issues during your pregnancy, consult your medical professional for proper testing, diagnosis, and treatment. Untreated thyroid disease during pregnancy may cause serious complications including pre-eclampsia.

Recommendations:
Cedarwood · Fennel
Idaho Blue Spruce
Myrtle · Sacred Frankincense

Topical:
- Apply 2-4 drops diluted 50:50 on temples, in clavicle notch (over thyroid), and behind ears 2-4 times daily as needed.
- Place a warm compress with 1-2 drops of chosen oil on the back.

URINARY TRACT INFECTION (UTI)

Urinary tract infections and inflammation known as cystitis are caused by bacteria that travel up the urethra. This disorder is more common in women because of their shorter urethra.

Recommendations:
Cistus · Juniper · Lemon
Melissa · Mountain Savory
Myrrh · Oregano · Spikenard
Tea Tree (Melaleuca Alternifolia)
Thyme

Topical:
- Dilute 50:50 and apply a few drops on location 3-6 times daily.
- Dilute 2-4 drops of Melrose, Purification, or other oil and use in a warm compress over bladder 1-2 times daily.
- Receive a Raindrop Technique 3 times weekly.
- First Week: Use Myrrh, Thyme, Mountain Savory, Palo Santo, and Inspiration and follow with a hot compress.

Ingestion & Oral:
- Take 1 capsule with desired oil 2 times daily.
- Put 2-3 drops of oil in a spoonful of Blue Agave, Yacon Syrup, maple syrup, coconut oil, milk, etc.
- Put the desired amount of oils in a glass of rice milk, almond milk, goat milk, carrot juice, NingXia Red, or even water and then drink it.
- Use K&B tincture (2-3 droppers in distilled water) 3-6 times daily. K&B helps strengthen and tone weak bladder, kidneys, and urinary tract.
- Take ½ teaspoon of AlkaLime daily, in water only, 1 hour before or after meal.
- Drink unsweetened cranberry juice and sweeten with honey, Yacon Syrup, Blue Agave, or maple syrup.
- Drink 4 liters of purified water daily.

UTERINE CARE

Natural hormones will change during pregnancy. Postpartum, you may need to give your uterus the best recuperation for future fertility.

Recommendations:
Clary Sage · Fennel
Fennel Vitality · Lady Sclareol
Melrose · Sage
SclarEssence · Thieves
Thieves Vitality

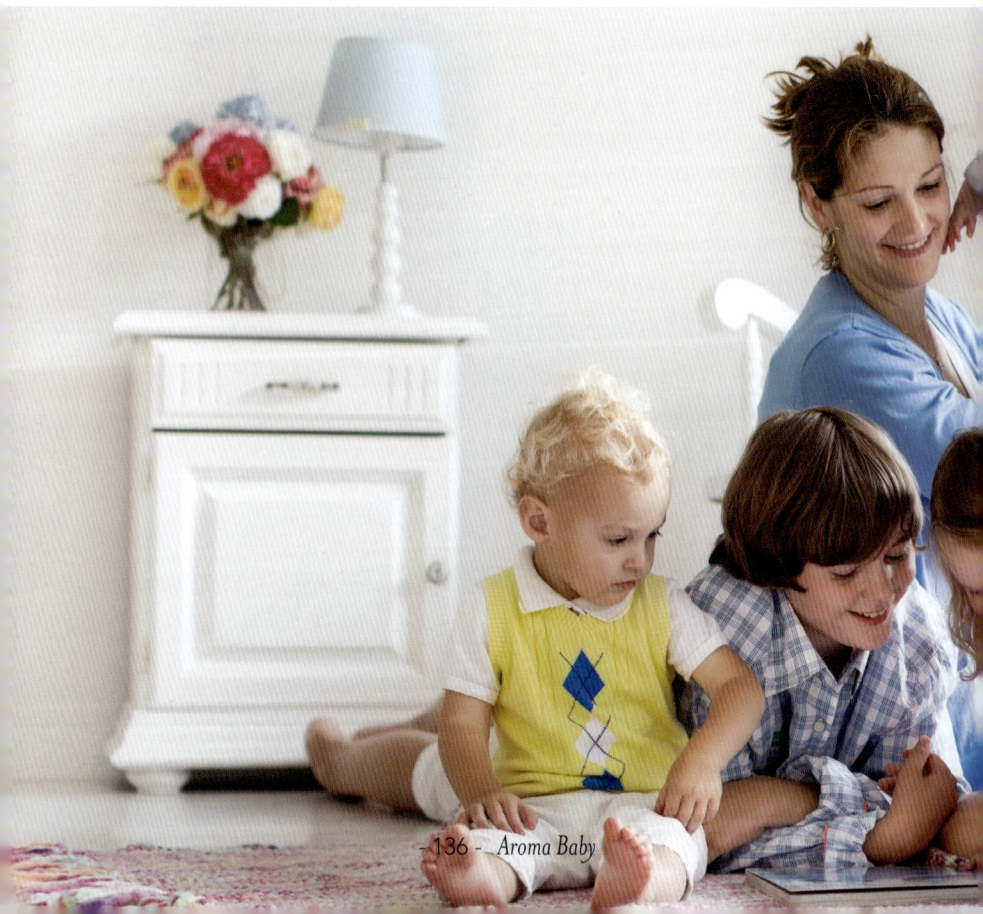

Inhalation:

- Diffuse your choice of oils for ½ hour every 4-6 hours or as desired.
- Put 2-3 drops of your chosen oil in your hands and rub them together, cup your hands over your nose, and inhale throughout the day as needed.
- Put 8-10 drops of oil on a cotton ball or tissue and put it in an air vent in your house, vehicle, hotel room, etc.
- If diffusing while sleeping, set your timer for the desired length of time for automatic shut off.

Topical:
- Apply a hot compress containing Melrose on the stomach.
- Massage 2-4 drops of Thieves blend neat on the soles of the feet.

Ingestion & Oral:
- Take 1 capsule with desired oil 2 times daily.
- Put 2-3 drops of oil in a spoonful of Blue Agave, Yacon Syrup, maple syrup, coconut oil, milk, etc.
- Put the desired amount of oils in a glass of rice milk, almond milk, goat milk, carrot juice, NingXia Red, or even water and then drink it.
- Colon and liver cleanse: ICP, ComforTone, Detoxzyme, Essentialzyme, JuvaPower

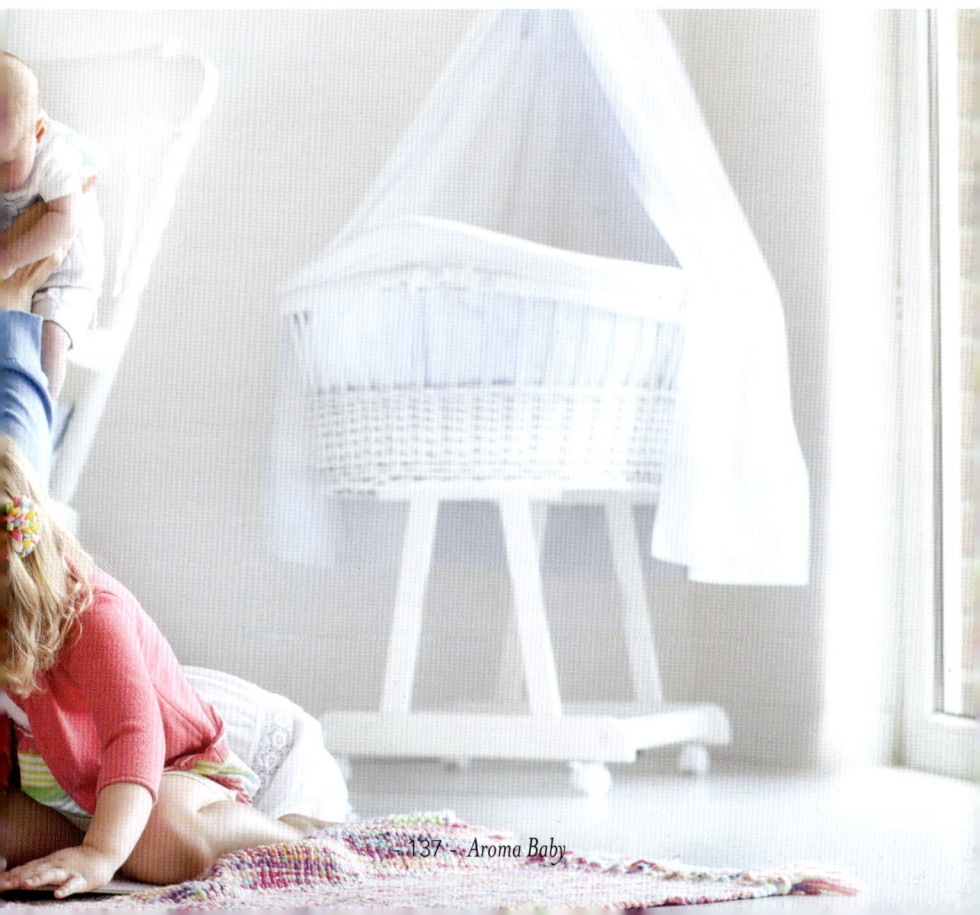

WATER BIRTH

Preparing for a water birth should only take place under the direction of a medical professional.

Topical:
Add 1–3 drops of undiluted essential oils directly to bath water. If more essential oil is desired, mix the oil first into bath salts or a bath gel base before adding to the bath water.

YEAST INFECTIONS

Vaginal yeast infections are just one symptom of systemic fungal infestation. While the yeast infection can be treated locally, the underlying problem of systemic candidiasis may still remain, unless specific dietary and health practices are used.

Vaginal Yeast Infection Blend
- 7 drops Melaleuca Alternifolia
- 5 drops Mountain Savory
- 2 drops Myrrh

Retention
- Mix an 80:20 ratio (8 parts chosen essential oil to 2 parts V-6 Vegetable Oil Complex), put 1-2 tablespoons on a tampon, and insert into the vagina daily for internal infection.
- Alternate approach: Douche with 1 tablespoon Thieves Fresh Essence Plus Mouthwash overnight 3 times a week. If it stings a little, dilute with a little V-6 Vegetable Oil Complex.

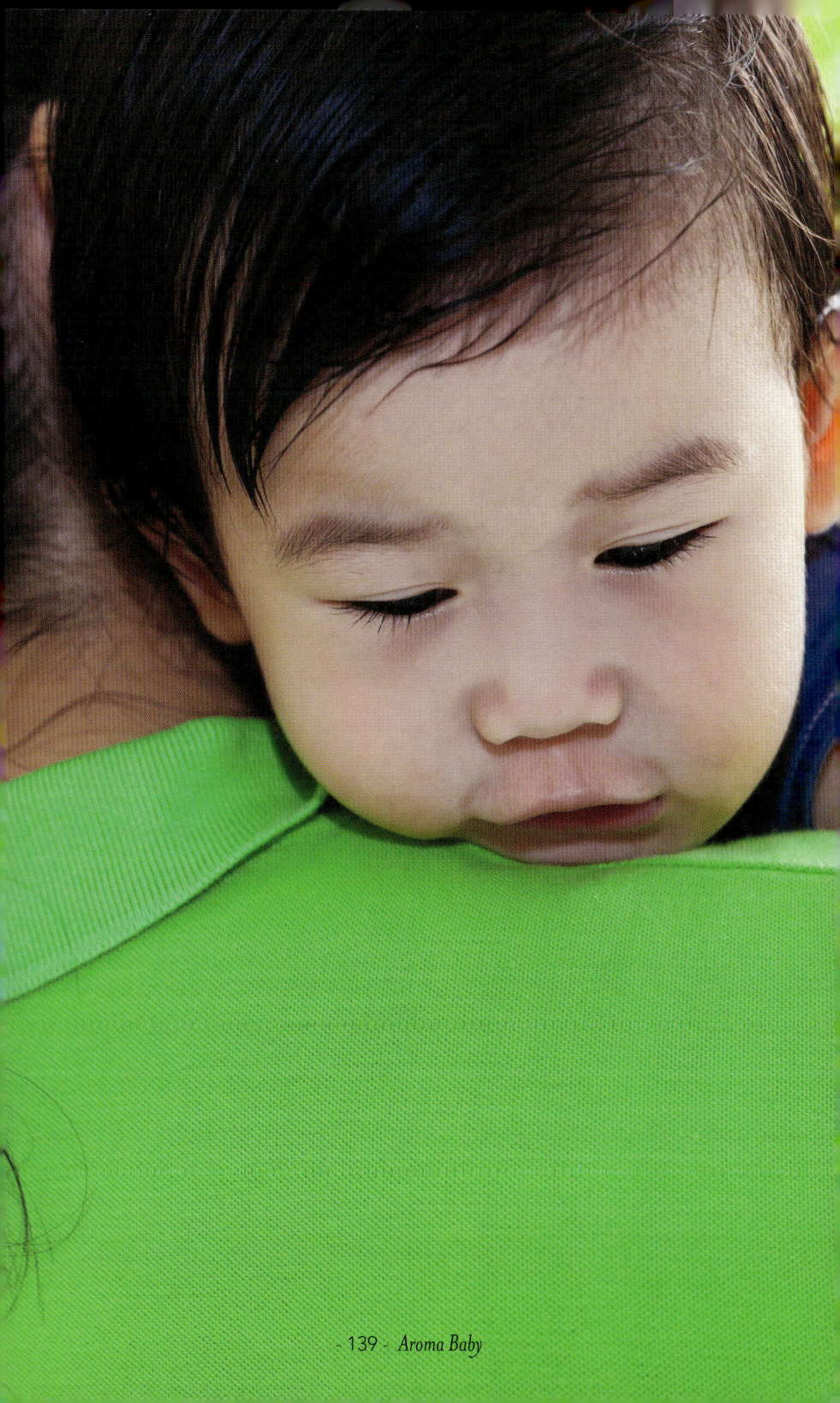

My favorites...

My favorites...

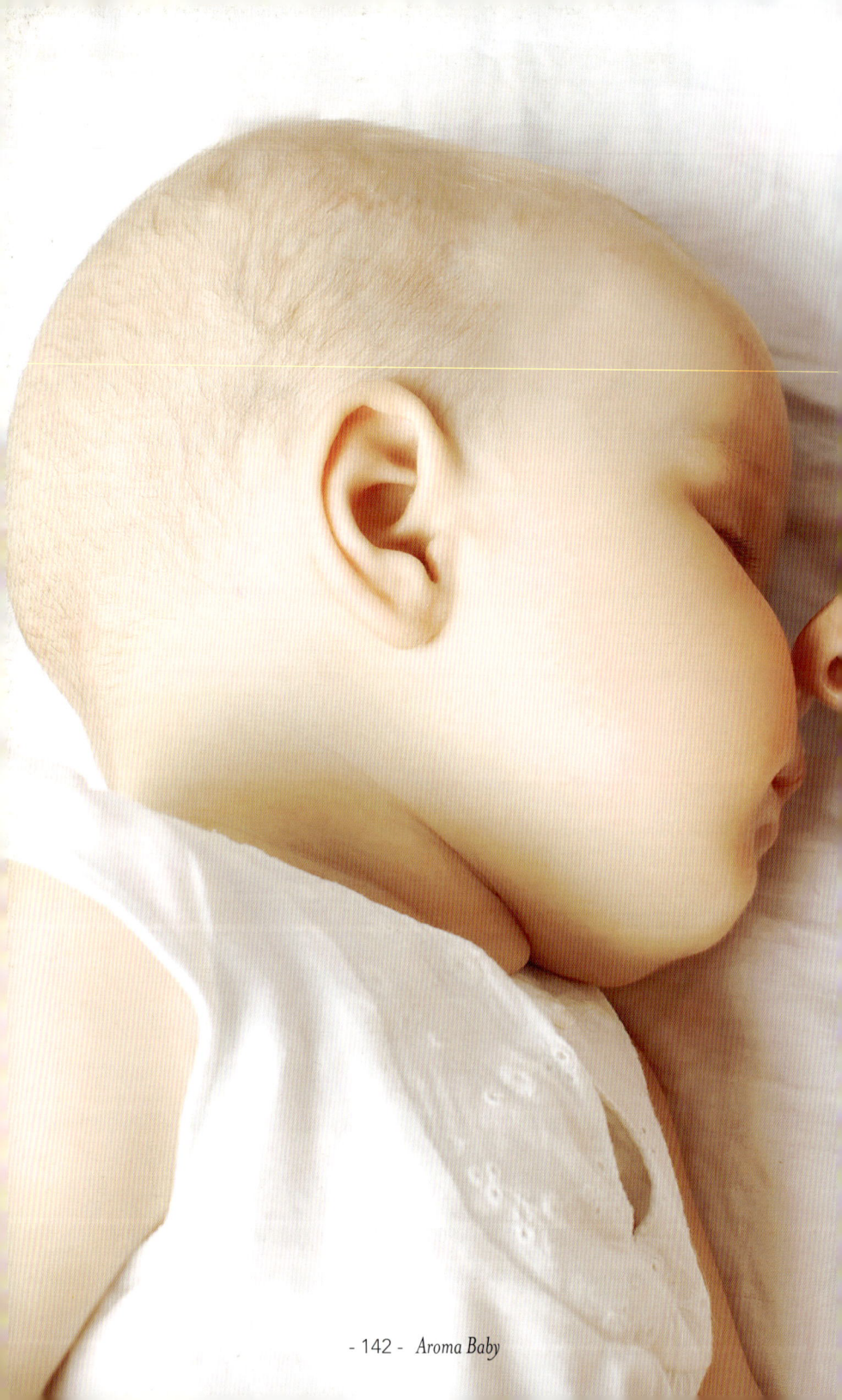

CONDITIONS: INFANTS

For the use of essential oils here, children are considered infants up until 24 months. Infants will readily absorb oils through their feet. However, they also tend to put their feet (and their hands) in their mouths, so be sure to keep this in mind. This is the most delicate time for them, so be sure to take great care as you use the different singles and blends. Remember, dilute the oils first to establish your baby won't have any reactions. Once you know how they respond, gently lower the dilution.

ACNE

Topical:
- Apply 4-6 drops diluted 50:50 to forehead, crown of the head, soles of the feet, lower abdomen, and lower back 1-3 times daily.
- Dab 1-2 drops on blemishes twice daily.

Recommendations:
Lavender
Lemon · Melrose

BATHING
(FOR BABY'S GENTLE SKIN)

Topical:
- Only use the mildest forms of bathing gels.
- Dilute 1-3 drops in KidScents Bath Gel.

Recommendations:
Gentle Baby
KidScents Bath Gel
Lavender

BOILS

Topical:
- Dab 1-2 drops diluted 50-50 on blemishes twice daily.

Recommendations:
Lavender
Lemon · Melrose

CHICKEN POX

Topical:
- Dab 1-2 drops diluted 50-50 on sores twice daily.
- Spray LavaDerm as needed to stop itching.

Recommendations:
Lavaderm
Lavender · Melrose

CIRCUMCISION

Topical:

- Dab 1-2 drops diluted 50-50 on tender areas twice daily.
- Spray LavaDerm as needed to stop inflammation.

Recommendations:
LavaDerm · Lavender
Melrose · Rose
KidScents Tender Tush

COLIC

Topical:

- Use a warm compress with Roman Chamomile to apply to stomach area.
- Add 1 drop Copaiba to 1 tablespoon of V-6 carrier and rub on baby's back.

Recommendations:
Copaiba
Roman Chamomile

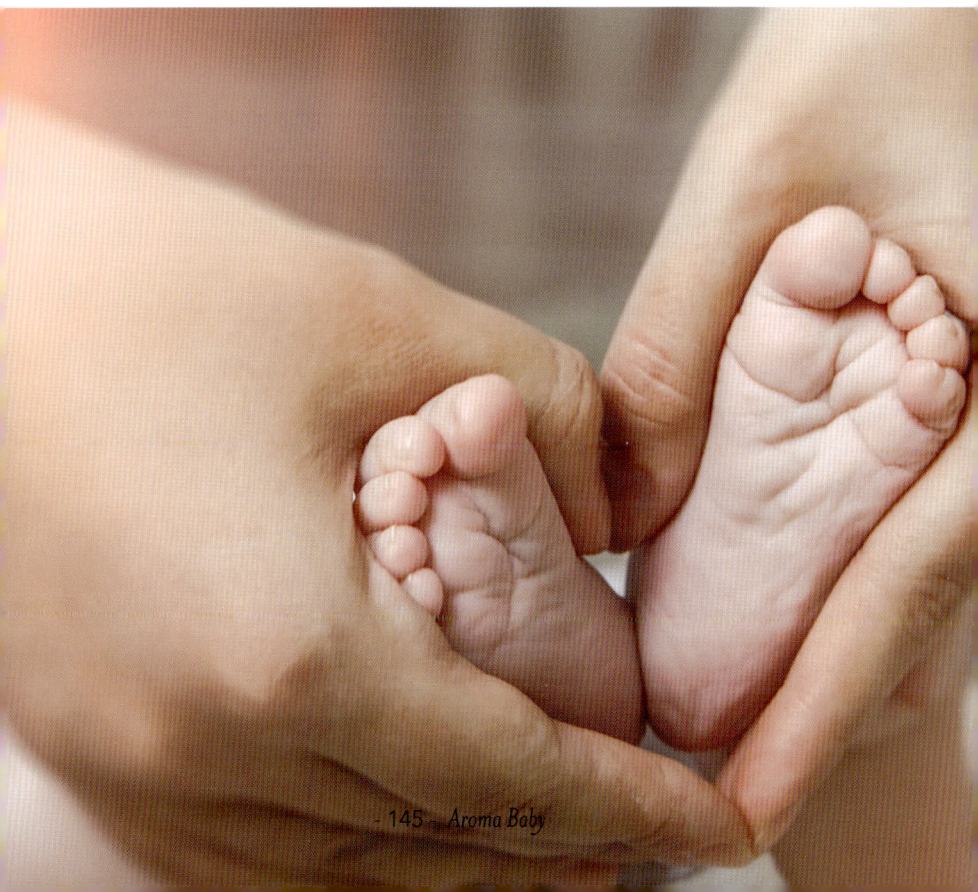

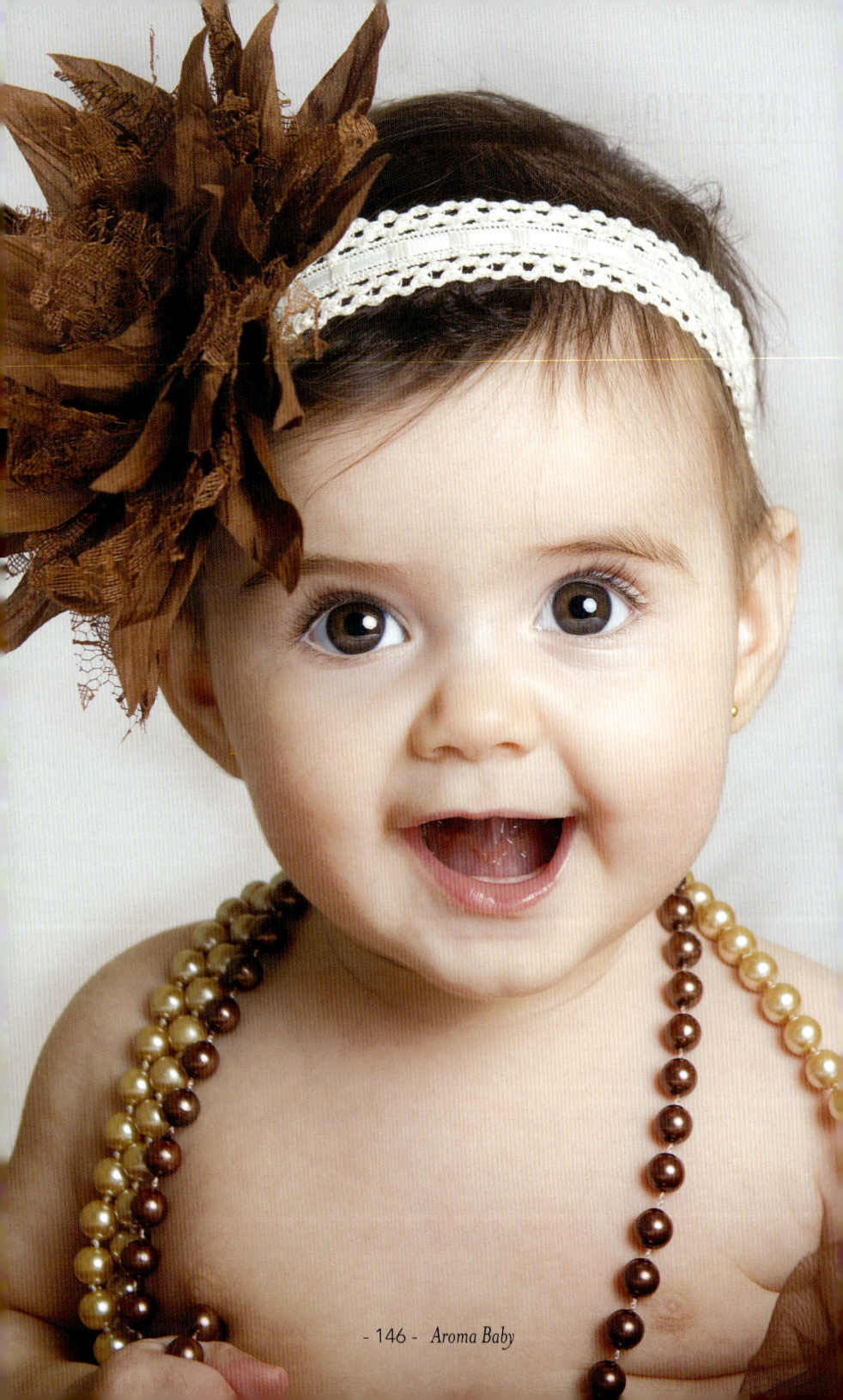

CONGESTION

Topical:
- Dilute 1-2 drops in 1 teaspoon of carrier and apply to shoulders, back, and neck.
- Dilute 1 drop Thieves in 1/2 teaspoon and apply to feet.

Recommendations:
Cedarwood
Lemon · Myrtle
Pine

CONJUNCTIVITIS (PINK EYE)

Topical:
- If lactating, drop 1 drop of expressed milk in each affected eye.
- Dilute 1 drop Melrose and Lavender each in 2 drops of V-6. Gently dab around the eye bone and socket area without getting it in your baby's eye.

Recommendations:
Lavender
Melrose

CONSTIPATION

Topical:
- Dilute 1-2 drops in 1 teaspoon of carrier and apply to baby's belly or abdomen.
- Dilute 1 drop in 1/2 teaspoon and apply to feet.

Recommendations:
Ginger
Lavender

COUGH

Inhalation:
- Diffuse your choice of oils for 20 minutes every 4-6 hours or just before bedtime.

Topical:
- Dilute 1-2 drops in ½ teaspoon carrier and dab across the chest. Cover with a onesie or shirt.

Recommendations:
Copaiba · Lavender
Lemon · Myrtle
Peace & Calming
Purification

CRADLE CAP
(SEBORRHEIC DERMATITIS)

Topical:
- Dab 1-2 drops diluted 50-50 on affected area twice daily.
- Dilute 1-2 drops in Rose Ointment and apply to affected area twice daily.

> Recommendations:
> Lavender · Lemon
> Melrose
> Rose Ointment

DIAPER RASH

Avoid products with Talc or mineral oil. Create your own baby powder out of cornstarch and essential oils. Use recommended essential oils below at a ratio of 10 drops per ounce/two tablespoons.

> Recommendations:
> Gentle Baby
> Kidscents Tender Tush
> Lavender
> Rose Ointment

Topical:
- Dab 1-2 drops diluted 50-50 on affected area twice daily.
- Dilute 1-2 drops in Rose Ointment and apply to affected area twice daily.

DIARRHEA

Topical:
- Dab 1-2 drops diluted 50-50 on abdominal area.

> Recommendations:
> Copaiba
> Lavender

DISINFECTION

Topical:

- Spray Thieves Spray as needed in baby's room to disinfect surfaces.
- Apply 1-2 drops of Thieves Vitality to disinfect pacifiers, bottles, and teething toys. Rinse and air dry.
- Dampen a clean paper towel. Add 2-3 drops to moist paper towel. Wring it gently to evenly distribute oil. Wipe surfaces.

Recommendations:
Thieves
Thieves Spray
Thieves Vitality

EAR INFECTION

Topical:

- Dilute 1-2 drops in ¼ teaspoon of carrier oil. Dip a cotton ball apply to all outer surfaces of the ear and behind the ear.
- Apply to baby's feet twice daily.

Recommendations:
Cedarwood
Lavender · Melrose

ECZEMA / DERMATITIS

Topical:

- Dilute 1-2 drops in ¼ teaspoon of carrier oil. Apply to affected areas.

Recommendations:
KidScents Tender Tush
Lavender · Melrose

EYE HEALTH

Topical:

- Add 1-2 drops to a cotton ball. Dab the bridge of the nose and the eye bone area, avoiding any contact with your baby's eye.

Recommendations:
Lavender

FEVER (OF UNKNOWN ORIGIN FUO)

Fever is most concerning for infants under 3 months. If fever exceeds 100.4°, seek immediate medical attention. If your infant is over 3 months and the fever lasts more than 24 hours, seek immediate medical attention. If fever is present with rash, difficulty breathing or swallowing, or your baby seems less than alert, seek immediate medical attention.

Recommendations:
Lavender
Lemon · Melrose

Topical:
- Dab 1-2 drops diluted 50-50 on bottoms of the feet twice daily.
- Apply 1-2 drops diluted 50-50 on bottom of the spine.

FUSSY

Babies may be fussy for any number of reasons. This is when your baby seems fussy without any apparent cause.

Recommendations:
Joy · Lavender
Peace & Calming

Inhalation:
- Apply to cotton ball and wave within inhaling distance.
- Diffuse for 20 minutes in baby's room, particularly before bedtime.

Topical:
- Dab 1-2 drops diluted 50-50 to feet and back of the neck.

GROUP BETA STREP

This type of bacteria is common and harmless in most adults with normal immune systems. However, it can cause life-threatening infections in infants.

Recommendations:
Thieves · Valor
Valor II

Topical:
- Dab 1-2 drops diluted 50-50 on feet to help prevent infection.

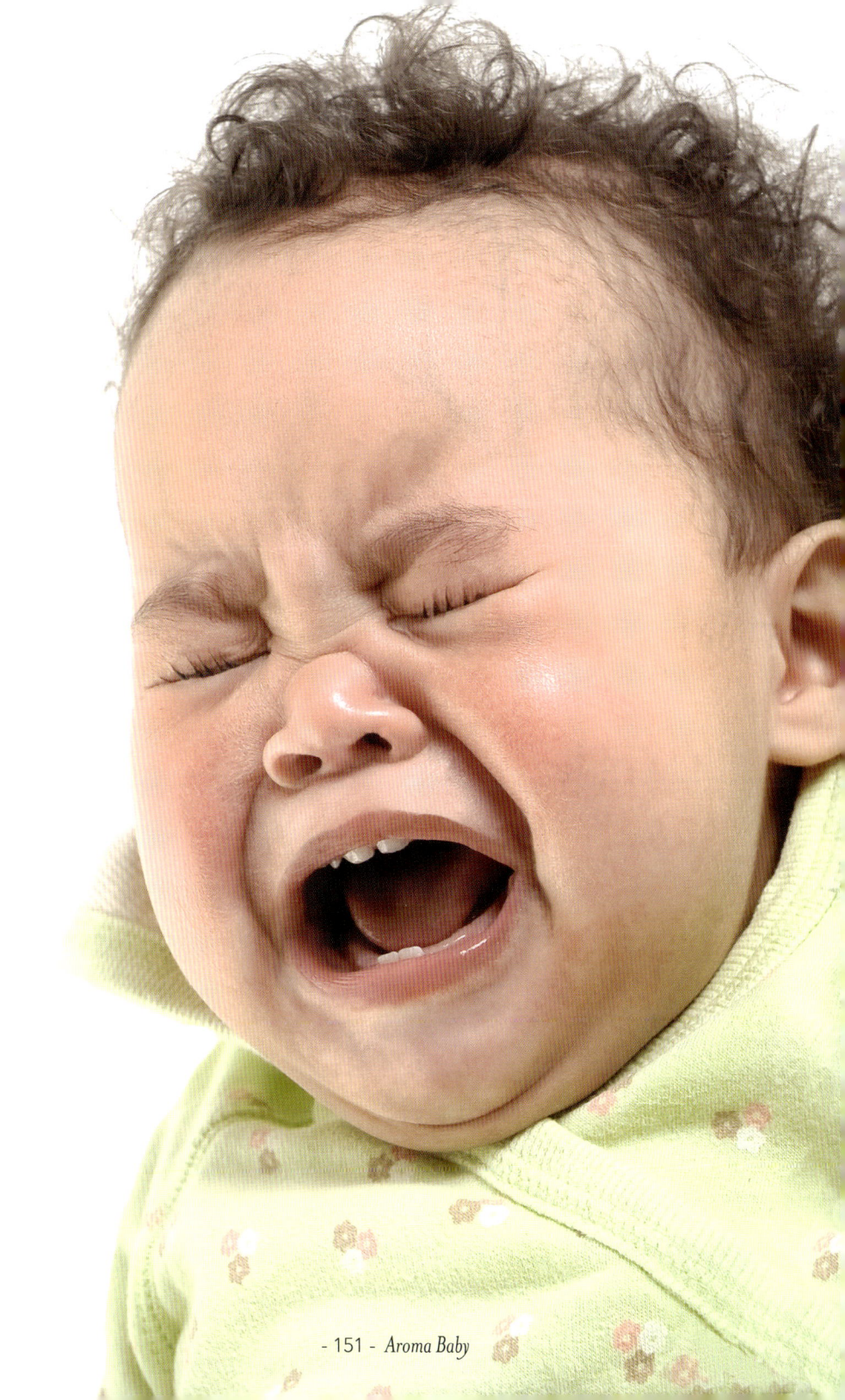

HAND-FOOT-MOUTH DISEASE
(COXSACKIEVIRUS A16)

This causes mouth sores, rash, blisters, and fever.

Topical:
- Dab 1-2 drops diluted 50-50 on feet four times daily.
- Dab 1-2 drops diluted 50-50 on spine twice daily.

> *Recommendations:*
> *Melrose · Lavender*
> *Purification*
> *Mountain Savory*
> *Thieves*

HIVES

Topical:
- Dilute 1-2 drops in ¼ teaspoon of carrier oil. Apply to affected areas.

> *Recommendations:*
> *KidScents Tender Tush*
> *Lavender · Melrose*

INDIGESTION

Topical:
- Use a warm compress with Roman Chamomile to apply to stomach area.
- Add 1 drop Copaiba to 1 tablespoon of V-6 carrier and rub on baby's back.

> *Recommendations:*
> *Copaiba · Lemon*
> *Roman Chamomile*

INSECT BITES

Topical:
- Dab 1-2 drops diluted 50-50 on affected area every three hours.

> *Recommendations:*
> *Purification*
> *Roman Chamomile*

INSECT REPELLENT

Topical:
- Dilute 5 drops of each in a 4-ounce spray bottle of distilled water. Shake well and mist the exposed areas.
- Dampen a clean paper towel. Add 2-3 drops Purification to moist paper towel. Wring it gently to evenly distribute oil. Wipe exposed skin areas.

Recommendations:
Peppermint
Purification

ITCHING

Topical:
- Dab 1-2 drops diluted 50-50 on affected areas as needed.

Recommendations:
KidScents Tender Tush
Lavender
Rose Ointment

JAUNDICE

Infant jaundice is relatively common, especially in preterm babies. The baby's liver isn't mature enough to filter bilirubin in the bloodstream. Most cases that need treatment respond well to noninvasive therapy.

Recommendations:
Geranium
Lemon · Orange

Topical:
- Dab 1-2 drops diluted 50-50 on feet twice daily.
- Allow your baby to have 10 minutes of indirect sunlight daily.

POISON IVY/OAK/SUMAC

Topical:
- Dab 1-2 drops diluted 50-50 on affected areas 2 to 4 times daily.

Recommendations:
Gentle Baby
Kidscents Tender Tush
Lavender
Peace & Calming

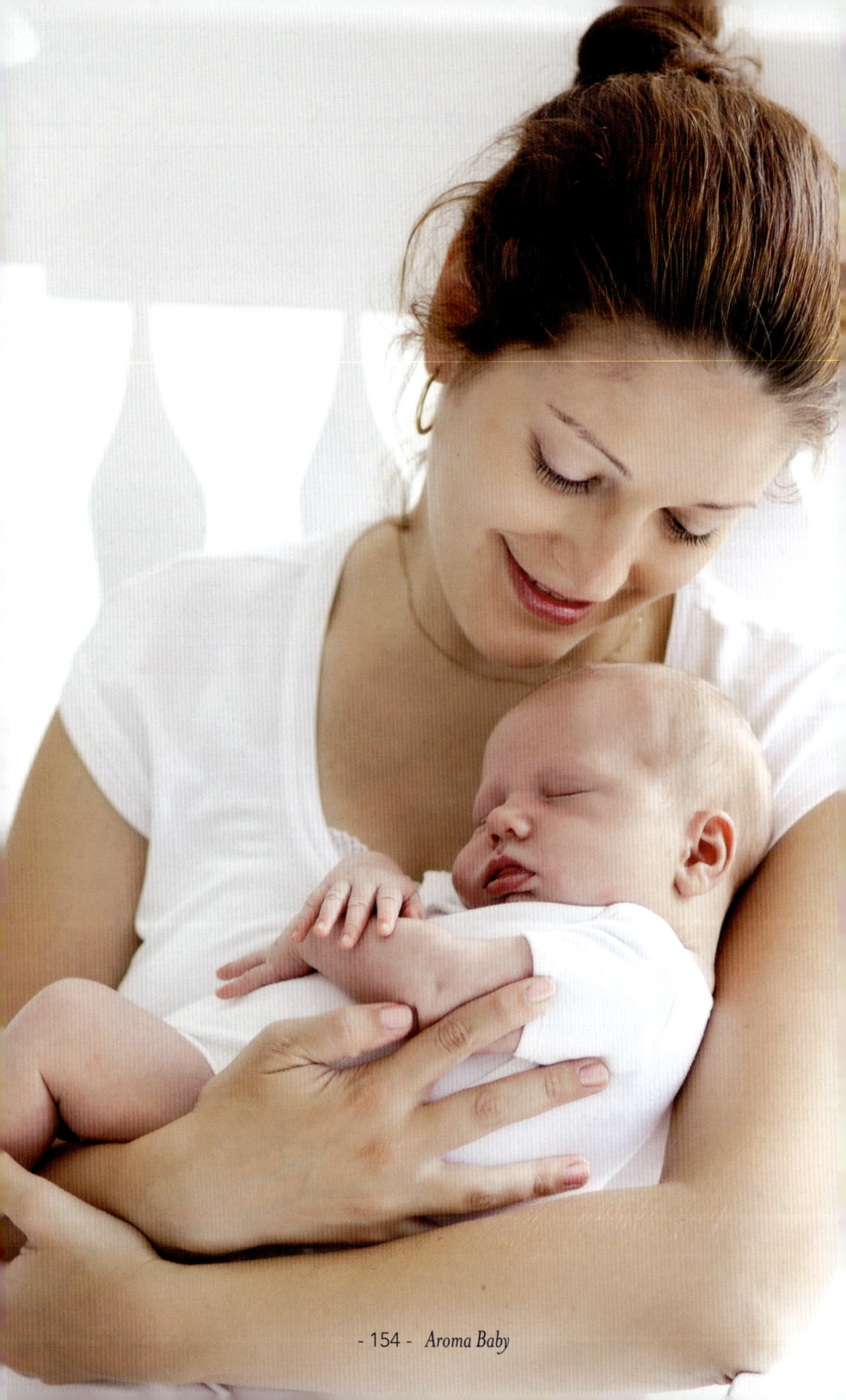

RESPIRATORY TRACT INFECTION

Inhalation:
- Diffuse your choice of oils for 20 minutes every 4-6 hours or just before bedtime.

> Recommendations:
> Copaiba · Frankincense
> Myrtle · Peace & Calming
> Ravintsara

Topical:
- Dilute 1-2 drops in ½ teaspoon carrier and dab across the chest. Cover with a onesie or shirt.

SKIN CARE

Topical:
- Dab 1-2 drops diluted 50-50 on affected areas as needed.

> Recommendations:
> KidScents Tender Tush
> Lavender · Melrose

TEETHING

Topical:
- Dab 1-2 drops diluted 50-50 on sore areas twice daily.

> Recommendations:
> Copaiba
> Frankincense Vitality
> Orange Vitality

THRUSH

- Dab 1-2 drops diluted 50-50 on your clean finger or cotton swab and gently swab your baby's mouth every 3 hours.

> Recommendations:
> Geranium · Lavender
> Melrose
> NingXia Red

UMBILICAL CORD STUMP

Keep the stump clean and dry. During the healing process, it's normal to see a little blood near the stump. Much like a scab, when the cord stump falls off, a little bleeding might occur. However, contact your baby's doctor if the umbilical area oozes pus or the surrounding skin becomes red and swollen.

Recommendations:
Frankincense
Geranium · Myrrh
Rose Ointment

Topical:
- Dab 1-2 drops diluted 50-50 on the umbilical cord stump.
- Dab 1-2 drops diluted 50-50 to areas around the navel for one week after the stump falls off.

YEAST INFECTIONS

- Dab 1-2 drops diluted 50-50 on your clean finger or cotton swab and gently swab your baby's mouth every 3 hours.

Recommendations:
Geranium
Lavender · Melrose
NingXia Red

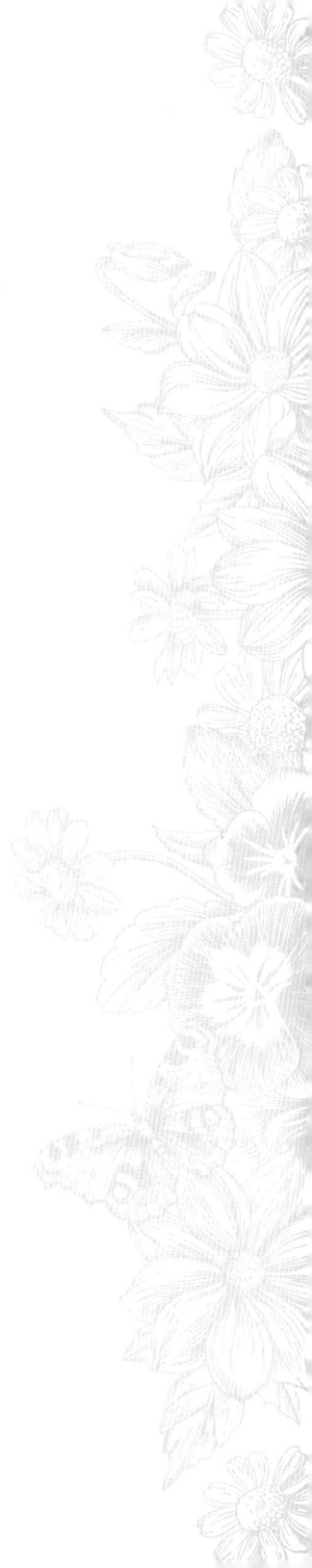

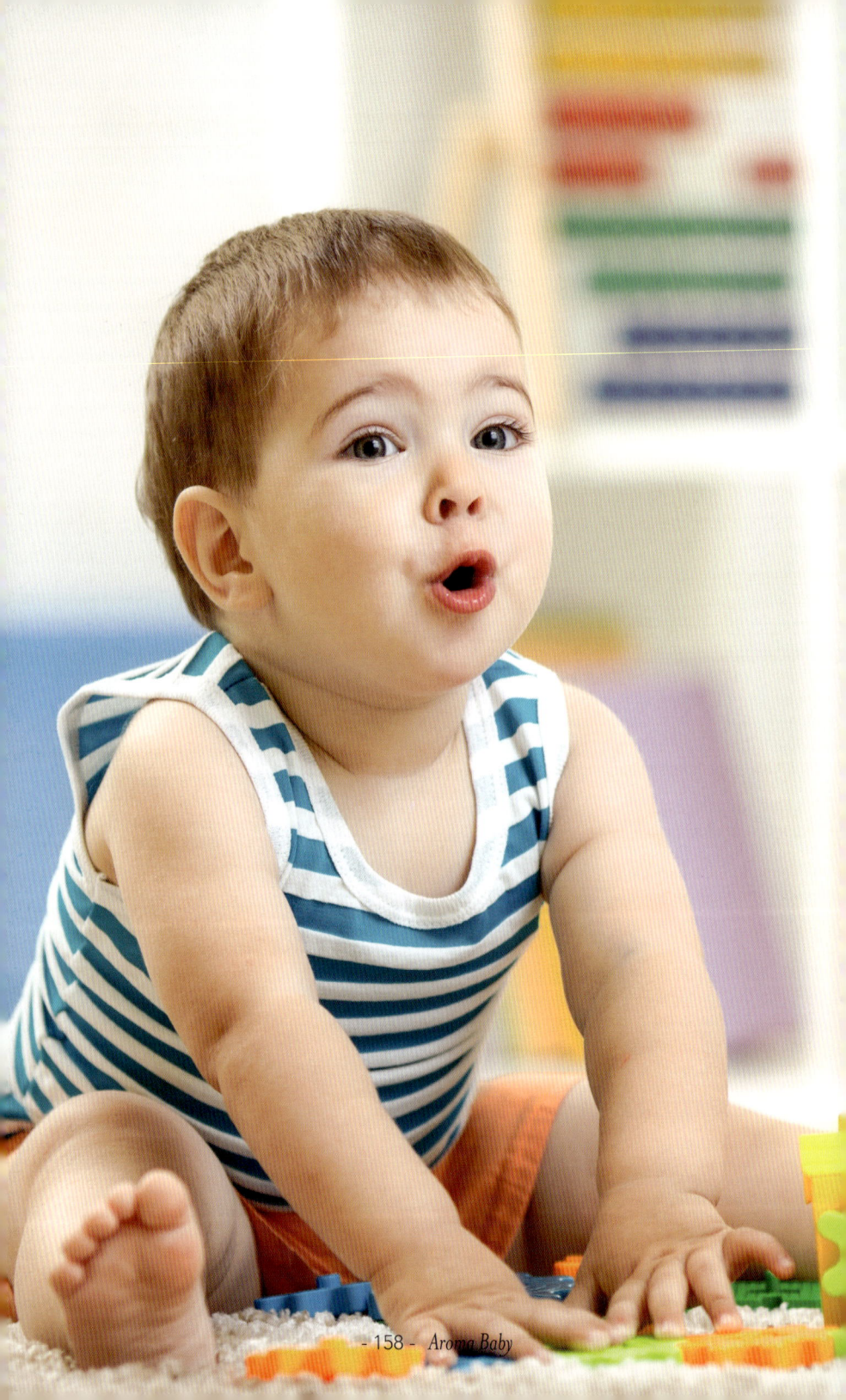

KIDSCENTS® BATH GEL

KidScents Bath Gel is a safe and gentle formula with a neutral pH balance perfect for young skin. This gel contains MSM (a natural form of sulfur that promotes healthy skin), aloe vera, a mix of antioxidant vitamins and botanicals, and pure Lemon and Cedarwood essential oils. KidScents Bath Gel contains no mineral oils, synthetic perfumes, artificial colorings, or toxic ingredients.

> **Directions:** Apply a small amount of KidScents Bath Gel to washcloth or directly to the skin. Rub gently, then rinse.

KIDSCENTS® LOTION

KidScents Lotion is safe, gentle, and pH neutral, ideal for young skin. It contains MSM, shea butter (with natural UV protection), aloe vera, wheat germ oil, almond oil, antioxidant vitamins, and essential oils. KidScents Lotion contains no mineral oils, synthetic perfumes, artificial colorings, or toxic ingredients.

KIDSCENTS® SHAMPOO

KidScents Shampoo contains the finest natural ingredients for gently cleansing children's delicate hair. A mild formula designed to provide the perfect pH balance for children's hair, KidScents Shampoo contains MSM (a natural sulfur compound known to strengthen hair), aloe vera, chamomile, and other herbs and vitamins. KidScents Shampoo contains no mineral oils, synthetic perfumes, artificial colorings, or toxic ingredients.

KIDSCENTS® TENDER TUSH

KidScents Tender Tush is a gentle ointment designed to protect and nourish young skin and promote healing. Formulated with natural vegetable oils and pure essential oils, the ointment soothes dry, chapped skin and offers protection for delicate skin. KidScents Tender Tush is also great for expectant mothers who are concerned about having stretch marks. Directions: Apply liberally to diaper area as often as needed to help soothe diaper rash, redness, or irritation.

KIDSCENTS® SLIQUE™ TOOTHPASTE

KidScents Slique Toothpaste is a safe, natural alternative to commercial brands of toothpaste. Formulated with Slique Essence and Thieves essential oil blends, this toothpaste gently cleans teeth and tastes great without synthetic dyes or flavors. Slique Essence is antibacterial, antifungal, a lipid regulator, and a glucose regulator. Thieves is antiseptic and antimicrobial and combats plaque-causing microorganisms.

KidScents Slique Toothpaste is perfect for children of all ages, and it makes a great training toothpaste for children during the crucial first years while they develop their primary teeth. Calcium carbonate, baking soda, and xylitol are used as tooth and gum health agents. This is a most amazing blend of highly antiviral, antiseptic, antibacterial, and anti-infectious essential oils.

Directions: Brush teeth thoroughly after meals or at least 2 times daily.

Caution: Keep out of reach of children. Store in a cool, dry place. Use caution to keep KidScents Slique Toothpaste out of children's eyes.

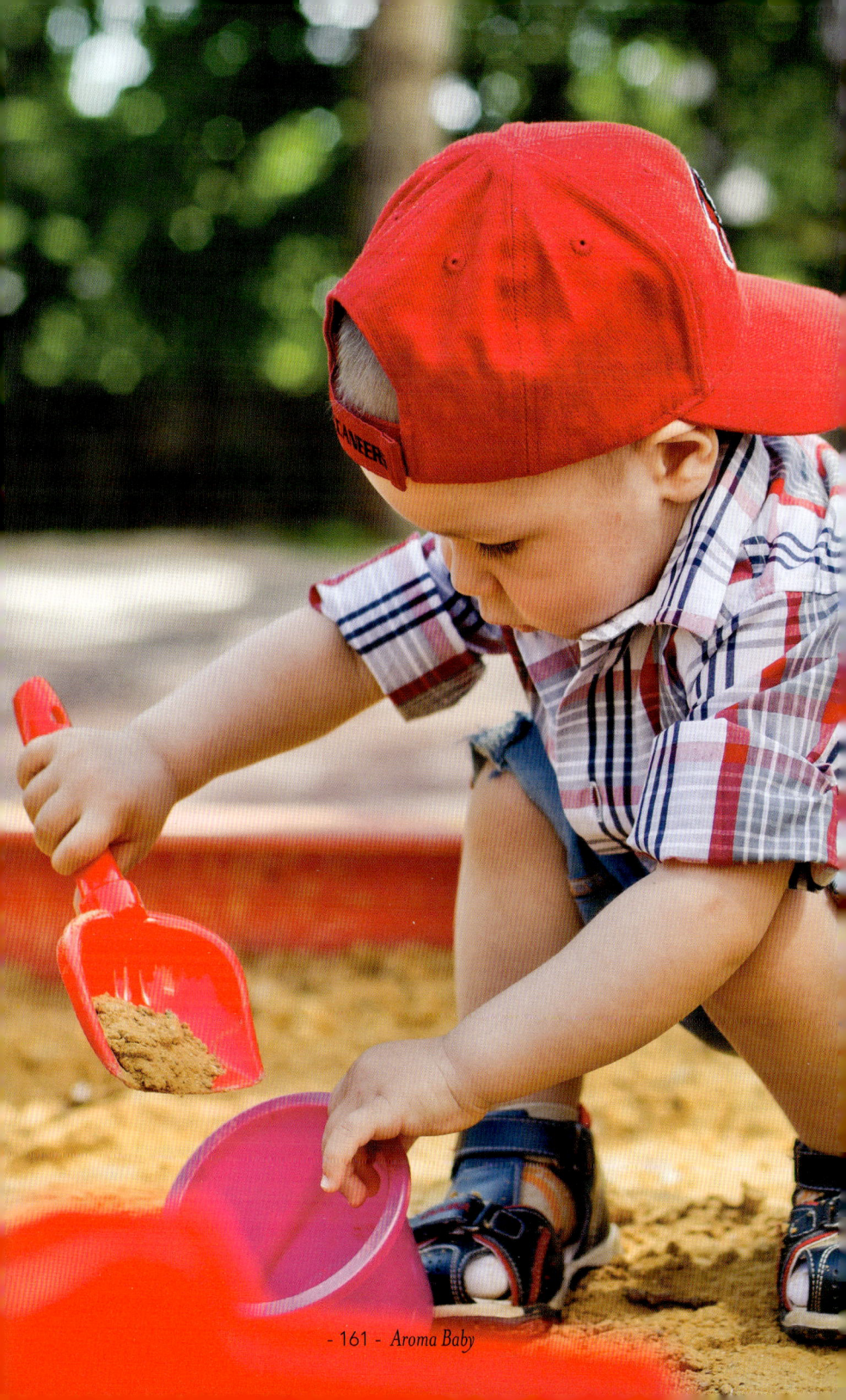

KIDSCENTS® MIGHTYVITES™

KidScents MightyVites are great-tasting, chewable multivitamin tablets, perfect for children's developing bodies, including increased immune function, brain development, and bone and joint health. Made with NingXia wolfberry (Lycium barbarum), KidScents MightyVites contain superfruits, plants, and vegetables that deliver the full spectrum of vitamins, minerals, antioxidants, and phytonutrients in their whole, synergistic, and easily-absorbable form. KidScents MightyVites come in two flavors, orange cream and mixed berry.

Directions: Children ages 6–12 years old, take 3 chewable tablets daily prior to or with meals.

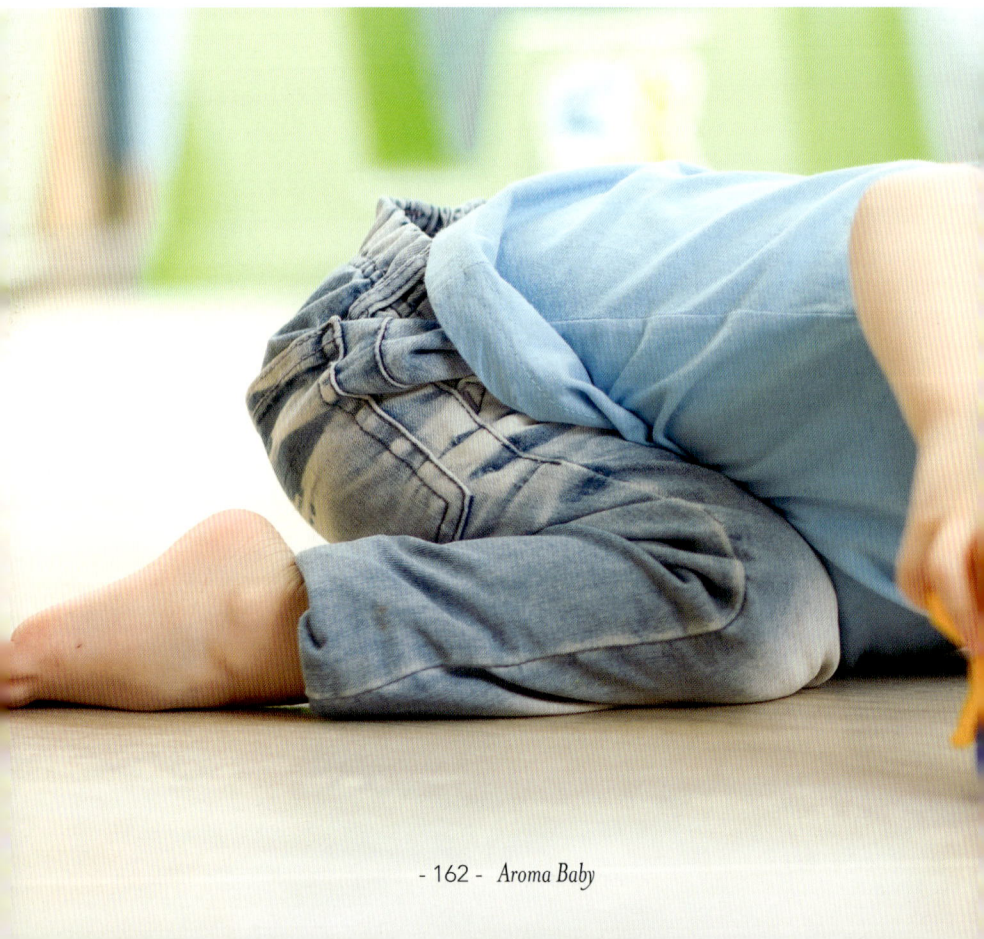

KIDSCENTS® MIGHTYVITES™ Orange Cream Flavor

KIDSCENTS® MIGHTYVITES™ Wild Berry Flavor

KIDSCENTS® MIGHTYZYME™

KidScents Mightyzyme is a special formulation containing nine different digestive enzymes and other nutrients designed to support healthy digestion in children. KidScents Mightyzyme also aids in the relief of occasional symptoms, including fullness, pressure, bloating, gas, pain, or minor cramping that may occur after eating.

Directions: Take 1 tablet 3 times daily prior to or with meals.

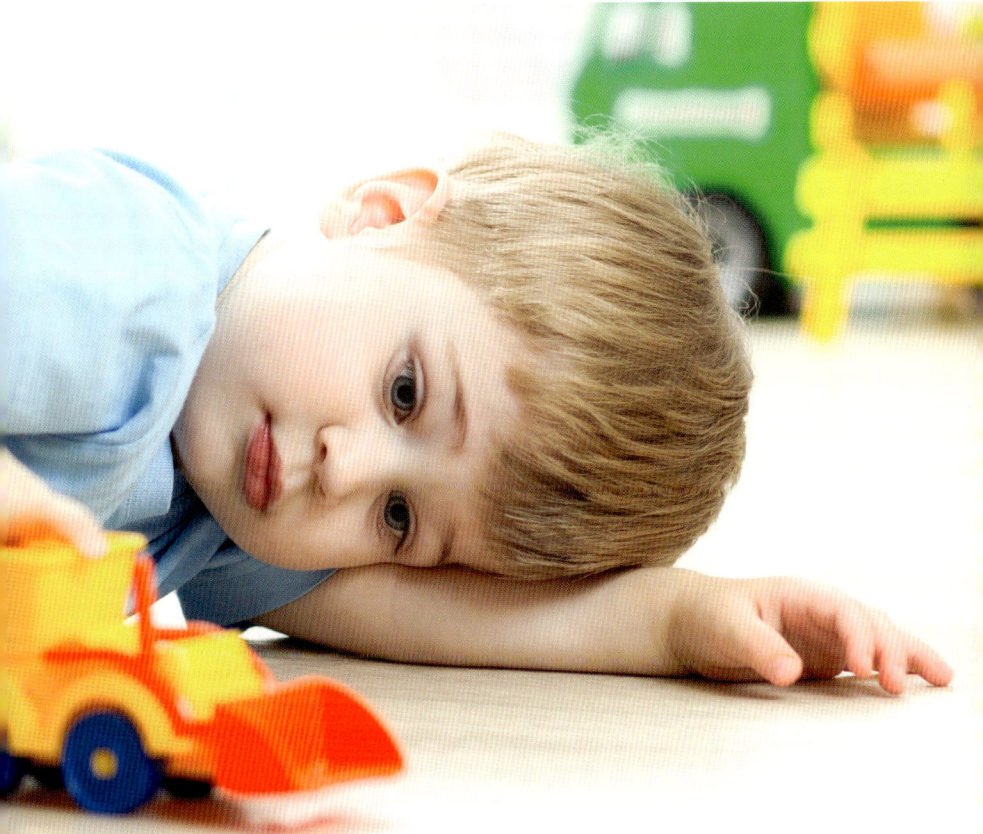

My favorites...

My favorites...

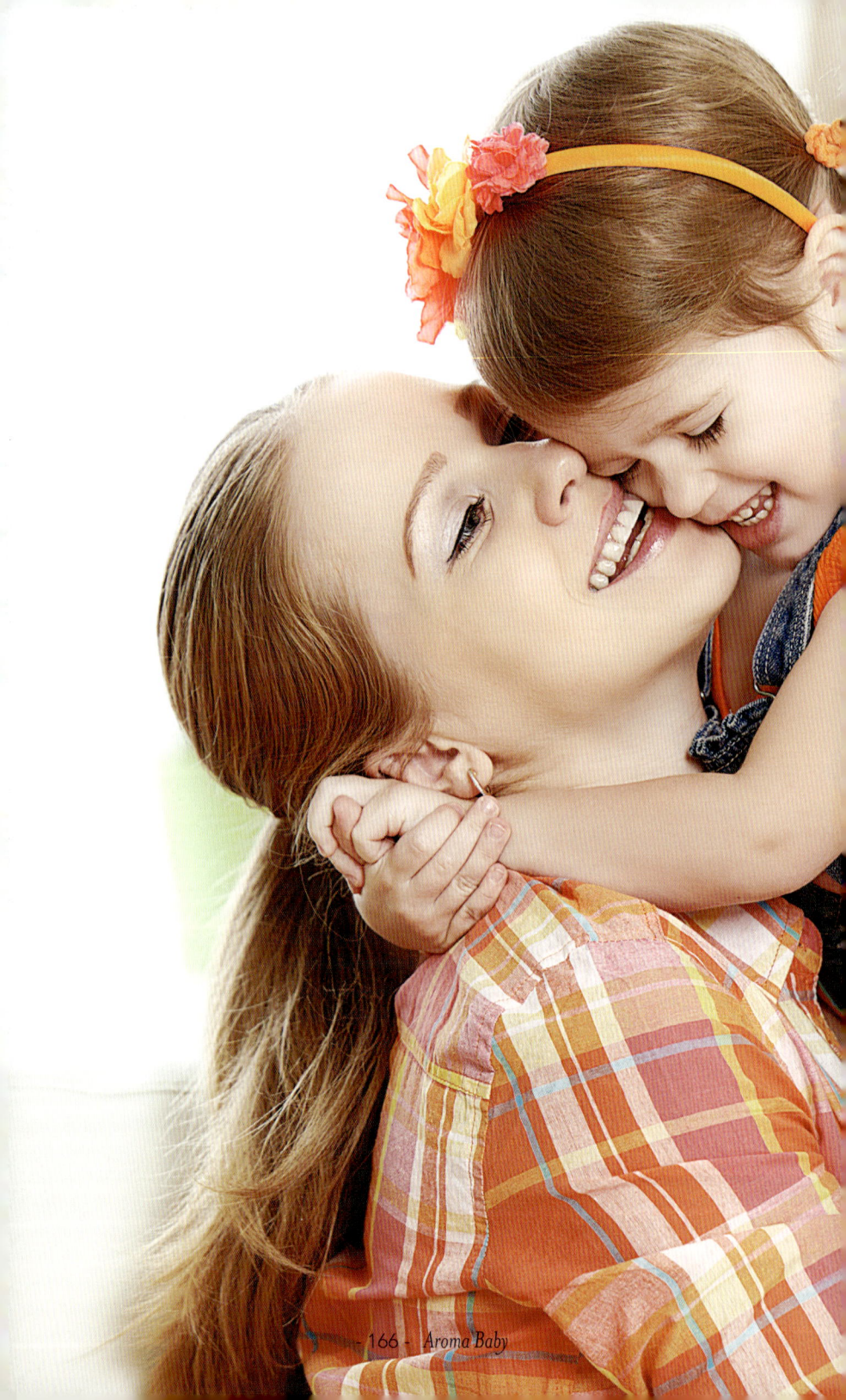

CONDITIONS: TODDLERS

For the purposes of the essential oil suggestions here, toddlers are children over 24 months. Their ability to process and absorb essential oils has progressed by this time so that they metabolize a little more and in slightly higher concentrations than infants. A toddler's feet are more developed and their body mass has increased as well as the surface area of their skin.

ALLERGIES

Inhalation:

- Place one drop on a cotton swab and gently swab the edge of the nostril.
- Diffuse your choice of oils for ½ hour every 4-6 hours or as desired.
- Put 2-3 drops of your chosen oil in your hands and rub them together, cup your hands over your nose, and inhale throughout the day as needed.
- Put 8-10 drops of oil on a cotton ball or tissue and put it in an air vent in your house, vehicle, hotel room, etc.
- If diffusing while sleeping, set your timer for the desired length of time for automatic shut off.

Recommendations:
Eucalyptus Radiata
Lavender
Lavender Vitality

Topical:

- Apply 1-2 drops diluted 50:50 just under your child's jawbone on right and left sides 4-8 times daily.
- You may also apply 2-3 drops on the Vita Flex points of their feet and hands.

Ingestion & Oral:

- Put 2-3 drops of Vitality line oil in a spoonful of Blue Agave, Yacon Syrup, maple syrup, coconut oil, milk, etc.
- Put the desired amount of oils in a glass of rice milk, almond milk, goat milk, carrot juice, NingXia Red, or even water and then drink it.

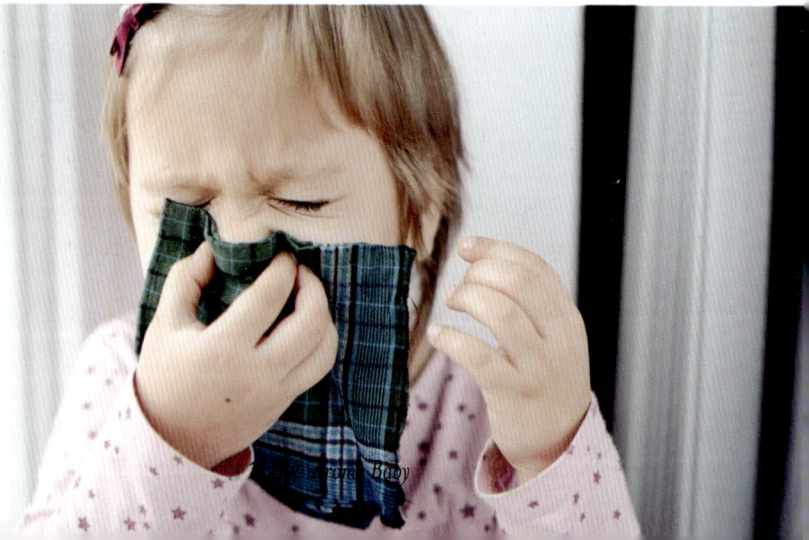

ASTHMA

Inhalation:

- Diffuse your choice of oils for 3-5 minutes or as often as it is comfortable.
- Put 8-10 drops of oil on a cotton ball or tissue and put it in an air vent in your house, vehicle, hotel room, etc.
- If diffusing while sleeping, set your timer for the desired length of time for automatic shut off.

Recommendations:
Dorado Azul · Eucalyptus Radiata
Sacred Frankincense
Ravintsara · Palo Santo

Topical:

- Apply 1-2 drops mixed with Ortho Ease, Relaxation, or Sensation massage oils on temples and back of neck as desired.
- You may also apply 2-3 drops on the Vita Flex points on the feet and hands.

AUTISM

Autism is a neurologically based developmental disorder that is four times more common in boys than girls.

Inhalation:

- Diffuse your choice of oils for 1 hour 4-6 times daily or as desired.
- Put 2-3 drops of your chosen oil in your hands and rub them together, cup your hands over your nose, and inhale throughout the day as needed.
- Put 8-10 drops of oil on a cotton ball or tissue and put it in an air vent in your house, vehicle, hotel room, etc.
- If diffusing while sleeping, set your timer for the desired length of time for automatic shut off.

Recommendations:
Brain Power · Cedarwood
Clarity · Eucalyptus Globulus
Frankincense · GLF
KidScents MightyVites
KidScents MightyZymes · Lavender
Melissa · NingXia Red · Patchouli
Peace & Calming · Sandalwood
Valor · Valor Roll-On · Vetiver

Topical:

- Apply 1-2 drops neat (undiluted) on temples and back of neck, as desired.
- Applying a single drop under the nose is helpful and refreshing.
- Massage 2-4 drops of oil neat on the soles of the feet just before bedtime.

BATHING

Topical:

- Only use the mildest forms of bathing gels.
- Dilute 1-3 drops in KidScents Bath Gel.

Recommendations:
Gentle Baby
KidScents Bath Gel
Lavender

BED WETTING

Topical:

- Apply Melrose diluted 50:50 over the area of the bladder before bedtime.
- You may also apply 2-3 drops on the Vita Flex points on the feet and hands.

Recommendations:
Melrose
Peace & Calming
Valor · Valor II

BOILS

Topical:

- Dab 1-2 drops diluted 50:50 on blemishes twice daily.
- Dab 1-2 drops neat on blemishes twice daily.

Recommendations:
Lavender
Lemon · Melrose

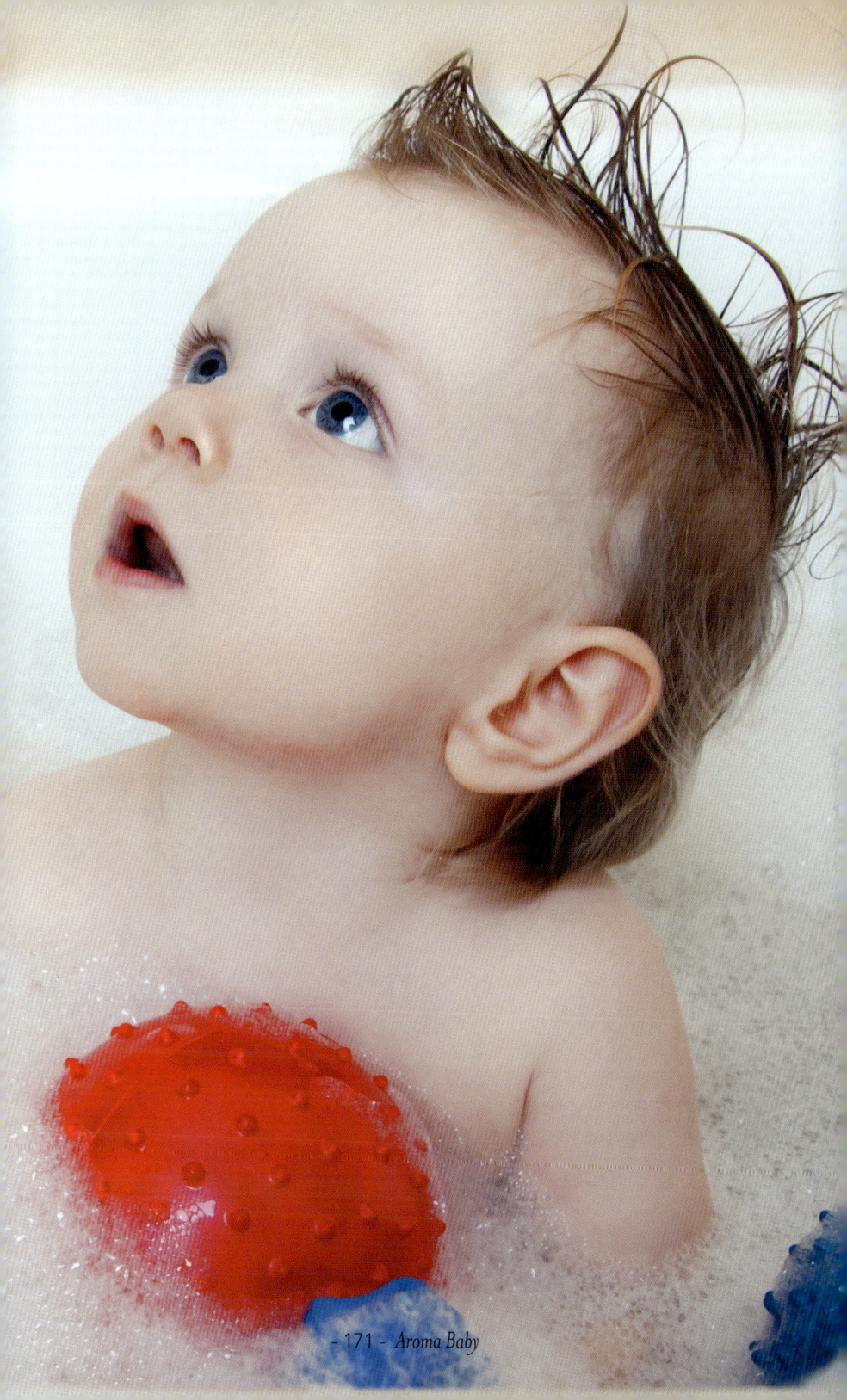

CHICKEN POX

Topical:
- Dab 1-2 drops diluted 50:50 on sores twice daily.
- Spray LavaDerm as needed to stop itching.

Recommendations:
LavaDerm
Lavender · Melrose

CONGESTION

Topical:
- Dilute1-2 drops in 1 teaspoon of carrier and apply to shoulders, back, and neck.
- Dilute 1 drop Thieves in 1/2 teaspoon and apply to feet.

Recommendations:
Cedarwood · Lemon
Myrtle · Pine

CONJUNCTIVITIS (PINK EYE)

Topical:
- Dilute 1 drop Melrose and Lavender each in 2 drops of V-6. Gently dab around the eye bone and socket area without getting it in your child's eye.

Recommendations:
Lavender
Melrose

CONSTIPATION

Topical:
- Dilute 1-2 drops 50:50 with carrier and apply to child's belly or abdomen.
- Dilute 1-2 drops 50:50 with carrier and apply to child's feet.

Recommendations:
DiGize · Ginger
Lavender · Peppermint

Oral:
- Give your child KidScents MightyVites and KidScents MightyZymes as directed.

COUGH

Inhalation:

- Diffuse your choice of oils for 20 minutes every 4-6 hours or just before bedtime.

Recommendations:
Copaiba · Lavender · Lemon
Myrtle · Peace & Calming
Purification

Topical:

- Dilute 1-2 drops in ½ teaspoon carrier and dab across the chest. Cover with a onesie or shirt.

DIAPER RASH

Avoid products with Talc or mineral oil. Create your own baby powder out of cornstarch and essential oils. Use recommended essential oils below at a ratio of 10 drops per ounce/two tablespoons.

Recommendations:
Gentle Baby
KidScents Tender Tush
Lavender · Rose Ointment

Topical:

- Dab 1-2 drops diluted 50:50 on affected area twice daily.
- Dilute 1-2 drops in Rose Ointment and apply to affected area twice daily.

DIARRHEA

Topical:

- Dilute 50:50 and apply 6-10 drops over stomach area 2 times daily.
- Apply a warm compress 1-2 times daily.
- Apply 1-3 drops on stomach Vita Flex points of feet.

Recommendations:
DiGize · DiGize Vitality · Ginger
Ginger Vitality · Lavender
Lavender Vitality · Peppermint
Peppermint Vitality · Rosemary
Rosemary Vitality

Ingestion & Oral:

- Take 1 capsule with desired Vitality line oil 2 times daily.
- Put 2-3 drops of Vitality line oil in a spoonful of Blue Agave, Yacon Syrup, maple syrup, coconut oil, milk, etc.
- Put the desired amount of oils in a glass of rice milk, almond milk, goat milk, carrot juice, NingXia Red, or even water and then drink it.

DISINFECTION

Topical:

- Spray Thieves Spray as needed in baby's room to disinfect surfaces.
- Apply 1-2 drops of Thieves Vitality to disinfect pacifiers, bottles, and teething toys. Rinse and air dry.
- Dampen a clean paper towel. Add 2-3 drops to moist paper towel. Wring it gently to evenly distribute oil. Wipe surfaces.

Recommendations:
Thieves · Thieves Spray
Thieves Vitality

EAR INFECTION

Topical:

- Dilute 1-2 drops in ¼ teaspoon of carrier oil. Dip a cotton ball apply to all outer surfaces of the ear and behind the ear.
- Apply to baby's feet twice daily.

Recommendations:
Cedarwood
Lavender · Melrose

ECZEMA/DERMATITIS

Topical:

- Dilute 1-2 drops in ¼ teaspoon of carrier oil. Apply to affected areas.

Recommendations:
KidScents Tender Tush
Lavender · Melrose

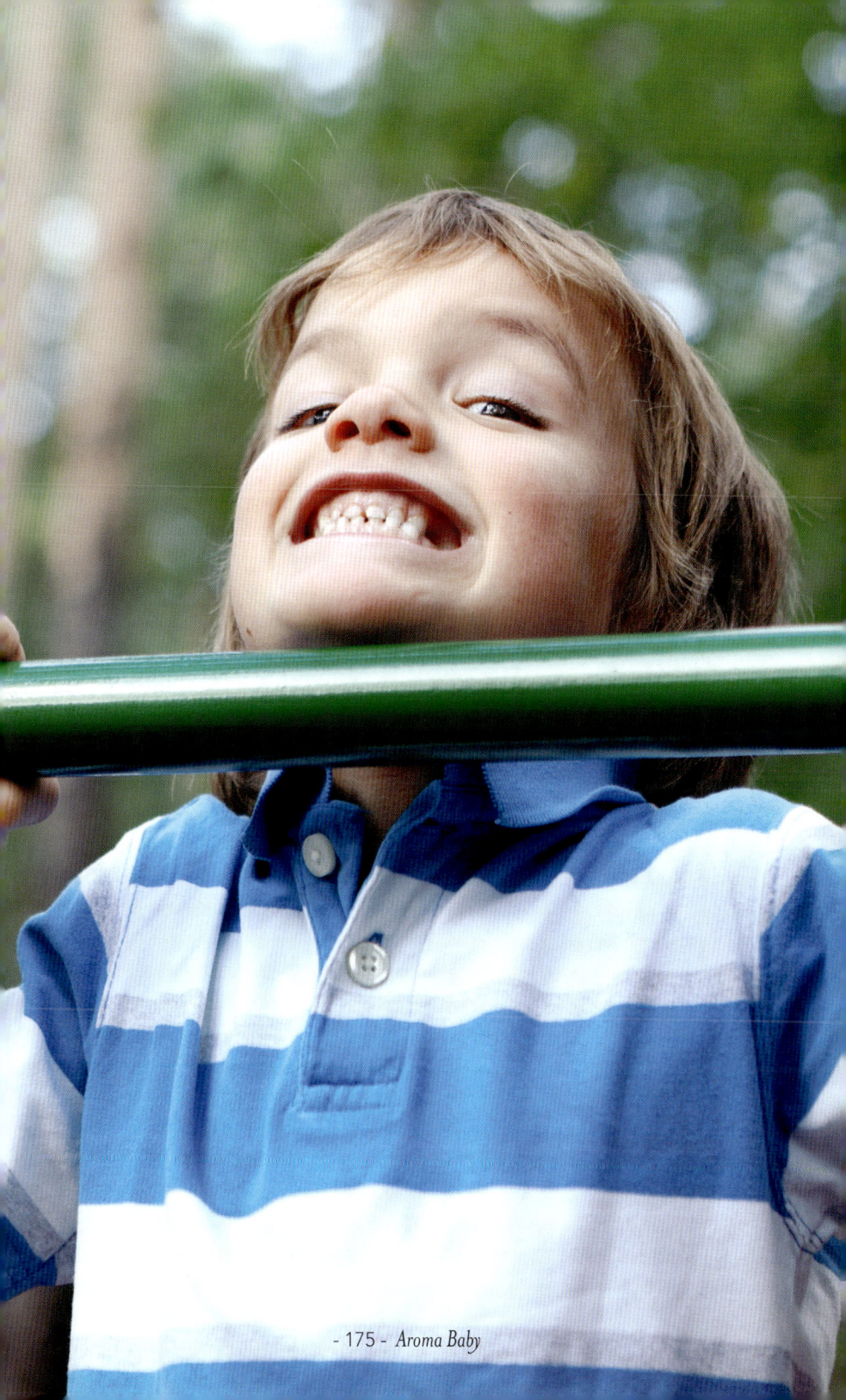

EYE HEALTH

Topical:

- Add 1-2 drops to a cotton ball. Dab the bridge of the nose and the eye bone area, avoiding any contact with your child's eye.

Recommendations:
Lavender

FEVER
(OF UNKNOWN ORIGIN 'FUO')

Topical:

- Dab 1-2 drops diluted 50:50 on bottoms of the feet every 4 hours.
- Apply 1-2 drops diluted 50:50 on bottom of the spine every 4 hours.
- Apply 1-2 drops of diluted Peppermint 50:50 on the navel every 4 hours.

Ingestion & Oral:

- Take one ounce of NingXia Red every two hours.

Recommendations:
Lavender · Lemon
NingXia Red · Peppermint
Thieves

HAND-FOOT-MOUTH DISEASE
(COXSACKIEVIRUS A16)

Topical:

- Dab 1-2 drops diluted 50:50 on feet four times daily.
- Dab 1-2 drops diluted 50:50 on spine twice daily.

Recommendations:
Melrose · Lavender
Purification
Mountain Savory
Thieves